THE MENOPAUSE DIET MINI MEAL COOKBOOK

THE MENOPAUSE DIET MINI MEAL COOKBOOK

Larrian Gillespie

Healthy Life
publications

Visit our website at
http://MENOPAUSEDIET.COM

Healthy Life Publications Inc.
264 S. La Cienega Blvd., PMB #1233
Beverly Hills, Calif. 90211
1-800-554-3335
1-310-471-2375
1-310-471-9041 FAX

Publisher's Cataloging-in-Publication
Provided by Quality Books, Inc.
Gillespie, Larrian
        The menopause diet mini meal cookbook : good food
for real women, naturally / Larrian Gillespie. – 1st ed.
        p. cm.
        Includes bibliographical references and index.
        ISBN: 0-9671317-1-5

        1. Menopause--Complications--Diet therapy--Recipes.
I. Title

RG186.G55 1999   618.1'750654
                                 QBI99-1103

First Healthy Life Trade Printing: November, 1999

Printed in the U.S.A.

10 9 8 7 6 5 4 3 2 1

The information found in this book is from the author's experiences and
is not intended to replace medical advice. The author does not directly or
indirectly dispense medical advice or prescribe the use of this nutritional
program as a form of treatment. This publication is presented for infor-
mational purposes only. Before beginning this or any nutrition program
you should consult with your physician.

Inside cover photo: Robert Cavalli, Still Moving Pictures
Book Design by: Barbara Hoorman

contents

chapter

dedication

To Alexian

Always my daughter
now too my friend

my mother
Dorothy Olive Gillespie

and my grandmother
Martha Tibeau

introduction

I was not "born to cook". Even my genes were against it. Though my mother was raised on a wheat farm in Assiniboia, Saskatchewan, Canada, she could present a turkey so undercooked I felt obligated to resuscitate it. They say some things skip generations, but whatever chromosome the cooking gene is on, it seems to have skipped a lot more than that in my family.

As a child raised in the San Fernando Valley, the only taste of decent cooking I ever had was when my grandmother would come to visit for the winter. I eagerly waited for her to bring out preserves she carefully brought down on the train, introducing me to gooseberries and red currants in exotic, quilted jars that glistened in the sunlight on the porch, where

My mother burned water which is why I was ten before I learned the fire alarm wasn't a kitchen timer

they were stored for those special occasions that never came. We actually ate something other than porridge for breakfast during her visits and I was in awe that scrambled eggs didn't have to contain the shells in order to provide a complete, nutritious meal. Let's face it—my mother burned water which is why I was ten before I learned the fire alarm wasn't a kitchen timer.

Dinner at home was more like attending a lynching than a family gathering. No one could decide upon a proper topic of conversation so everyone just shouted for as long as it took to divide up the spoils of the evening that were placed before them. Then silence would descend as we tried to identify parts even another chicken couldn't recognize. Some nights I prayed the oven could flush.

All this leads to why I am uniquely qualified to write this cookbook, which can turn anyone into a gourmet chef by my family standards. Simply put—I love food and enjoy everything about it! I recognize we, as menopausal mamas, have no time to waste in the kitchen when there is so much life to experience, so I have designed The Menopause Diet Mini Meals to be quick and delicious. You won't need a certificate from a cooking school to understand the recipes and I even provide a sample menu plan to get you started in the right direction. So go on...put on that apron and join me in becoming the healthiest women ever!

Larrian

You won't need a certificate from a cooking school to understand the recipes

chapter one
the making of a food surgeon

At the tender age of 5, after suffering from a medical scare that left me to believe I might only live a few years, I quietly told my parents I wanted to be a doctor. It was that simple. Now, 45 years later, I think of myself as a "Food Surgeon," dissecting nutrition labels instead of bodies, patching up recipes so they can fulfill their destiny—to help each of us live a healthy life. Even my kitchen, with all its knives in graduated, sharpened order, could sub as an operating room in the event of a disaster if it weren't for the floating dog hair and bird seed scattered on the floor.

As women entering menopause or barreling through it like a fire sale at Neiman Marcus, more than 50% of us have some degree of difficulty in breaking down carbohydrates, which can lead to a tangled web of insulin resistance, plaque formation, hypertension and heart attacks—the number one killer of women.[1] So why are we encouraged to eat a high carbohydrate diet?

The answer is simple: research on metabolism and digestion have only recently focused on the difference between the way men's and women's stomachs handle food. Unlike men, women add an extra hour onto digestion because of the influence of hormones on the rate at which our stomachs are able to move food from the upper portion, the fundus, to the lower or antral portion.[2,3] During menopause, this delay in emptying becomes even more pronounced, causing us to lose the normal feeling of fullness as the result of a slower rise in glucose and insulin.[4] Over time this causes our cells to become resistant to the glucose lowering effect of insulin, which leads to obesity and all the diseases related to simply being overweight.

In the last 10 years, research has focused on the fact that not all carbohydrates are created equal when it comes to bestowing a Buddha Belly on women in menopause. Using the glycemic index, a guide that describes the rise in your blood sugar after eating a meal, scientists have classified carbohydrate-containing edibles by their rate of absorption and digestion into low, moderate or high-glycemic foods. Just eating a bag of buttered, high-glycemic popcorn can induce a cascade of hormonal changes that leads to excessive hunger and overeating.[5]

Eating more protein than currently recommended can protect you from the cancer-stimulating effects of estrogen therapy

the menopause diet

In "The Menopause Diet" you will find an extensive discussion about the effect hormones have on our ability to gain and lose weight and what you can do to be the healthiest ever at this stage in your life. You will discover "The Menopause Diet" is not about dieting but living a lifestyle that improves your chances of surviving to 100 without the disability brought on by heart disease, diabetes and high blood pressure. But more importantly, you will understand why eating more protein than currently recommended can protect you from the cancer-stimulating effects of estrogen therapy.

protein kryptonite

By current nutritional standards, eating a diet higher in protein than carbohydrates has received a bad rep in today's press, but does it really deserve it? A closer look at the mechanisms behind estrogen metabolism may prove it can be your personal kryptonite against cancer caused by too much estrogen in your system.

The synthesis and breakdown of estrogen involves enzymes, called cytochrome P-450, in liver and fat cells but also your ovaries. A specific enzyme, estrogen-2-hydroxylase (E2OHase), converts estrone into a non-estrogenic metabolite that is excreted in urine. This enzyme is affected by drugs, body fat and protein in your diet.[6]

the bio-availability of estradiol

| Androstenedione (AD) | Estrone (E_1) | 2-hydroxyestrone ($2OHE_1$) | 2-methoxyestrone ($2MeOE_1$) |

| Testosterone (T) | Estradiol (E_2) | 16$\propto$-hydroxyestrone ($16OHE_1$) | Estriol (E_3) |

figure 1

The metabolite, 2-OHE, binds to and prevents activation of your estrogen receptors, especially in the uterus. Not so for 16-OHE, which attaches to the same receptor and increases the amount of available circulating estradiol. This can lead to breast cancer and systemic lupus erythematosus, an estrogen-dependent disease.[7,8]

Eating a protein rich diet can even increase the activity of your CP-450 enzymes. When individuals were fed a diet composed of 44% protein and 35% carbohydrates, there was a profound affect on the activity in the 2-OHE pathway, favoring estrogen deactivation.[9] Even a low fat diet can protect your tissue, shifting estradiol metabolism away from the 16-αhydroxylation pathway and towards the cancer-preventing 2-hydroxylation route.[10] It doesn't take a superman to understand that a diet composed of 40%

protein, 25% fats and 35% low-glycemic carbohydrates can send you leaping into the air with a single
bound if you take estrogen replacement therapy!

And if you're concerned that too much protein
can weaken your kidneys and your bones, think
again. When women with type 2 diabetes (non-
insulin dependent or NIDDM) eat high protein
diets, they actually decrease their blood sugar and put
less stress on their kidneys than women who eat a low
protein, high glycemic carbohydrate diet.[11] Worries
about making your body too acid are also
unfounded, as sugar and starch cause more acidosis
than eating protein.[12] It seems the arginine in protein
derived from chicken or beef actually protects your
kidneys' sensitive filtering units by increasing the
blood flow through more relaxed microarteries.[13, 14]
No one is suggesting you eat only protein, which can
cause your body to remodel the calcium content in
your bones. Instead, by including fruits and
vegetables, which are high in potassium in your daily
diet, you reverse any urinary calcium loss.[15] So don't
be afraid to eat more protein. It could be just the leg
you need to stand on.

sweet talk

Sugar and spice make everything nice, especially
when you use seasonings that contain chromium, a
nutrient that helps to maintain insulin sensitivity in
your tissues. Scientists have discovered that spices
such as cinnamon, tumeric, cloves, bay leaves and
fennel seeds can triple insulin's ability to sweep
glucose into your hungry cells.[16, 17] No wonder Greek,
Mexican and the nomadic cultures of North Africa
favor these spices in their cooking. You will find the
recipes in "The Menopause Diet Mini Meal
Cookbook" make extensive use of these flavor
accents. And don't be afraid to add a little sugar to
any of the recipes. Although I have designed the 250
calorie mini meals without the addition of sugar,

research has shown that sugar, when added to foods, has no additional effect on blood glucose levels than those of the sugar alone, and can prevent you from increasing your intake of fat and high glycemic carbohydrates.[18]

salt: the new luxury ingredient

It's reported in the Bible that God turned Lot's wife into a pillar of salt when she disobeyed His instructions not to look back at the destruction of Sodom and Gomorrah. Fortunately, I can promise no such disaster will befall you if you indulge in the new luxury ingredient of the millennium—natural sea salt. For several decades, salt has been blamed for a host of diseases, but suddenly, it's coming back into favor. Salt is every bit as essential to our health and survival as when we first shed those flippers and scales and emerged from the sea and migrated inland.

Salt wakes up the flavor in food and improves the taste of almost everything, allowing flavors to mature and come into harmony in a dish. Today you can purchase a selection of sea salts that can sparkle like the crown jewels when you scatter them over summer-ripe tomatoes or grind a few crystals over fish or pork. Afraid salt will make you blow up like a puffer fish in a whistling competition? Not to worry—elevated insulin levels and lower amounts of peripheral deiodination of thyroxine (T4) in your body are to blame.

the thyroid theory

Women in menopause, and especially post-menopausal women, can develop "subclinical hypo-thyroidism" detected by the presence of antibodies to the thyroid gland. Nearly 70% of women age 70 have subclinical hypothyroidism which is a risk factor for coronary heart disease.[19, 20] In a study of healthy middle-aged women, 26% were found to have unsuspected subclinical hypothyroidism identified by the presence of antibodies and higher thyroid stimulating hormone levels than women without antibodies.[21] However, the addition of iodine to salt may cause significant changes in someone who has subclinical hypothyroidism, even in small doses.[22] In Japan seaweed wraps, which come from kelp that is high in iodine, caused marked hypothyroidism among those who ate it daily.[23] So using salt with iodine may be tipping the balance in your thyroid function.

Using salt with iodine may be tipping the balance in your thyroid function

If you taste table salt, it has a bitter flavor due to the chemicals that are added along with the iodine, causing the zinc in your saliva to give it a metallic taste. In comparison, sea salt has a sweet taste. Try switching your salt to a natural sea salt that has not been treated with additional iodine. I bet you will find it takes very little to bring a new flavor balance to your food and your weight.

it's an egg-xaggeration

The egg may not be the cholesterol-raising culprit it was once believed, especially if you are already eating a low-saturated-fat diet. It seems diets high in carbohydrates impair your glucose tolerance and increase your triglyceride levels while reducing the good cholesterol in NIDDM individuals.[24] In fact, researchers are rethinking cholesterol's role in cardiovascular crimes. It seems people vary widely in their ability to metabolize cholesterol, and compensate for absorbed dietary cholesterol by decreasing the amount produced in the liver or by increasing the cholesterol excreted, along with bile, from the gallbladder. Even eating 21 eggs a week can't make cholesterol stick around in healthy, young women.[25] And if you want to protect your eyes, nothing can beat the humble egg yolk as the nutritional champ for levels of the carotenoids, lutein and zeaxanthin.[26] So try the omelette recipes in the book and remember–if the cholesterol don't stick ...you must acquit!

the chocolate diet

No, I'm not recommending your consume a diet based on chocolate, but including some in your weekly Menopause Diet Plan won't cause any harm. It seems cocoa butter contains stearic acid, which can actually drop your cholesterol levels.[27] Although it is a highly saturated fat, its melting point is above body temperature, making it less well absorbed. I myself am partial to a California product by Scharffen Berger that contains 70% cocoa butter, but in a pinch I have been known to munch on a Dove silky dark chocolate chunk or a Snickers bar, all of which have been tested and found to fall in the moderate range for raising your blood sugar levels.[28] If you want to see the full listing of foods tested to date, and their GI ratings, read "The Glucose Revolution: The Authoritative Guide to the Glycemic Index" by Miller and Wolever or connect to http://www.mendosa.com/gi.htm on the web. This site contains a wealth of information about the GI values of food and is constantly updated as new research becomes available.

the non-nutrient: fiber

Increasing fiber in your diet can help protect sensitive tissues from too long an exposure to active estrogens such as estrone and estradiol. It seems having a regular bowel movement reduces the time estrogens have to be reabsorbed from stool in the colon, which cuts down on the amount of circulating estrogen.[29] It can also keep your blood sugar in check while helping with weight loss. Women taking estrogen replacement therapy should focus on including fiber-rich foods in their diet, especially pears, apples and beans. I have included several recipes that make sure you obtain enough insoluble fiber to keep those hemorrhoids that were a gift from your child-bearing years in seclusion.

the stinking rose

Garlic and members of the onion family, such as leeks, shallots, chives and scallions, have been used to treat an array of ills since the dawn of civilization. Packed full of antioxidants, these foods can help protect against cancer, elevated cholesterol levels and strokes. They were even used to protect against food poisoning by the ancient Mesopotamians. I have used them liberally throughout "The Menopause Diet Mini Meal Cookbook" not only for their flavor, but to demonstrate how easy it is to make food your home pharmacy.

the menopause diet mini meal menu plan

After reading "The Menopause Diet," you should understand the importance of keeping the amount of food you eat at a single time to around 250 calories if you want to keep your blood sugar on an even track and burn calories efficiently.[30] And if you choose a diet that emphasizes vegetables, beans and fruit along with low-GI carbohydrates, protein and fat, you can send glucagon, the hormone that mobilizes stored fat, on a seek and destroy mission while preventing hunger attacks.[5] So let's look at a sample 7-day menu plan for someone who needs to eat 5 meals a day, or 1250 calories, and is taking estrogen replacement therapy.

Calories	Protein 40%	Fat 25%	Sat 10%	Carbs 35%
1250	500	312.5	125	437.5
1500	600	375	150	525
1750	700	437	175	612
2000	800	500	200	700

Now look at the number of grams that represents, remembering that 1 gram equals 9 fat calories but only 4 calories from protein or carbohydrates.

Calories	Protein Gm	Fat Gm	Sat Gm	Carb Gm
1250	125	34.7	14	109.3
1500	150	41	16	131
1750	175	48.6	19	153.4
2000	200	55	22	175

Not planning on taking estrogen? Then use a 35/25/40 ratio instead as discussed in The Menopause Diet. It's easy to customize The Menopause Diet plan to suit your particular choices, so let's take a look at my personal diet for a week. As you can see it's full of good food for real women.

day one

	Total	Meal	Calories
	Cal: 1362		
	Protein: 130 g	1. Connemara Irish oatmeal (p. 94)	304
	Carbs: 136 g		
	Fat: 37 g	2. Tuna and white bean salad (p. 35)	275
	Sat: 10 g		
		3. Calcutta chicken in spinach and yogurt sauce (p. 66)	235
		Winter fruit salad (p. 103)	76
		4. Fourth of July cottage cheese (p.136)	227
		5. Seared black scallops (p. 59)	138
		Chilled cantaloupe and mint soup (p. 50)	104

day 2

Meal	Calories	Total
		Cal: 1290
1. Bahian black bean chili (p. 95)	221	Protein: 125 g
		Carbs: 121 g
2. Fourth of July cottage cheese (p. 136)	227	Fat: 39 g
		Sat: 11 g
3. Cuban grilled skirt steak (p. 80)	159	
Leeks Nicoise (p. 87)	109	
4. Grilled chicken and		
mandarin orange salad (p. 31)	273	
5. Tu Tu Tun Lodge grilled salmon (p. 61)	250	
Kabocha squash with Tunisian flavors (p. 86)	49	

day 3

Meal	Calories	Total
		Cal: 1201
1. Smoked salmon with apples (p. 60)	237	Protein: 133 g
		Carbs: 78 g
2. Tuna dip (p. 130)	69	Fat: 38 g
Thai shrimp broth with lemongrass, chili		Sat: 7 g
and ginger (p. 49)	121	
3. Mussels in chipotle chili broth (p. 55)	178	
Moroccan orange salad (p. 33)	70	
4. Baked Basque cod (p. 62)	140	
Aztec zucchini (p. 82)	95	
5. Indian turkey cutlets (p. 70)	154	
Red lentil and tofu curry (p. 100)	137	

day 4

Total	*Meal*	*Calories*
Cal: 1225		
Protein: 119 g	1. Rogue River salmon omelette (p. 24)	186
Carbs: 106 g	Joel's asparagus bake (p. 84)	32
Fat: 39 g		
Sat: 11 g	2. Crab with spicy orange dressing (p. 29)	138
	Yogurt and nuts (p. 136)	161
	3. Lemon tarragon chicken (p. 71)	223
	Zucchini noodles with spicy tomato sauce	44
	(p. 90)	
	4. Strawberries with cassis, balsamic vinegar	
	and mint (p. 106)	180
	5. Sea bass with chili and saffron (p. 58)	261

day 5

Total	*Meal*	*Calories*
Cal: 1340		
Protein: 133 g	1. Fennel and lemon soup (p. 46)	150
Carbs: 110 g	Spiced fruit salad (p. 105)	107
Fat: 45 g		
Sat: 8 g	2. Shrimp salad (p. 34)	274
	3. Moorish spicy lamb kebabs (p. 76)	165
	Rosemary and lemon pinto beans (p. 98)	96
	4. Chicken, tofu and watercress stir-fry (p. 67)	159
	Stir-fried bok choy (p. 89)	86
	5. Herbed tomato juice (p. 139)	37
	Halibut with artichokes, zucchini	
	and tomatoes (p. 54)	208
	Tuscany eggplant (p. 85)	57

day 6

Meal	*Calories*
1. Rogue River salmon omelette (p. 24)	186
Smoky "virgin" mary (p. 142)	26
2. Cream of bell pepper soup (p. 43)	94
Shrimp with two mushrooms (p. 57)	165
3. Roasted turkey breast (p. 67)	70
Apple, walnut, grapes and celery salad (p. 38)	162
Fruit toddy (p. 138)	20
4. Sear-roasted halibut (p. 63)	237
5. Pork chops with chipolte marinade (p. 77)	175
Roasted peaches with cardamom (p. 108)	78

Total
Cal: 1216
Protein: 133 g
Carbs: 74 g
Fat: 45 g
Sat: 12 g

day 7

Meal	*Calories*
1. Breakfast protein shake	192
2. Tomato and pumpkin soup (p. 48)	110
Garbanzos with garlic and kale (p. 97)	122
3. Spicy beef with basil (p. 79)	217
Yellow tomato, watermelon and	
arugula salad (p. 104)	96
4. Eggplant dip (p. 133)	123
Tofu and veggies snack (p. 134)	54
5. Orange roughy with orange, caper and	
olive sauce (p. 52)	190
Balsamic roasted squash and apples (p. 83)	109

Total
Cal: 1216
Protein: 92 g
Carbs: 138 g
Fat: 39 g
Sat: 7 g

weekly average

Cal: 1265
Protein: 124 g (38%)
Carbs: 109 g (34%)
Fat: 40 g (28%)
Sat: 9 g (7%)

As you can see, it's all just a balancing act when you're trying to lose weight, so don't be afraid to put a little "wiggle" into your diet. It's what you take in over several days that counts, not each and every bite. Even the overweight steelworker in "The Full Monty" recognized "the less I eat...the fatter I get!" So do like his friend advised...just "stuff yourself and get thin" with The Menopause Diet Plan. In a way, you could say "The Menopause Diet" is not about the change of life, but rather having the time of your life making choices that can only lead to a healthier, more youthful you!

Part of the secret of success in life
is to eat what you like and
let the food fight it out inside.
~ Mark Twain ~

chapter two

table scraps
"throw away" cooking tips for
"The Menopause Diet"

• To conserve on oil, heat a pan dry on high heat until you can't hold your hand over the pan for longer than a count of three. Then add your oil and reduce the heat before adding your meat or vegetables. In this way the food will absorb the least amount of fat and won't boil in its juices.

• All dried herbs, including seeds, should be rehydrated before using in any recipes. To do this, dampen a paper towel and lay the herbs and spices on the towel and fold it over. After 5 minutes, remove the herbs from the towel and they are ready to use. This will improve the fragrance and flavor from your spices. If you are using seeds, such as coriander, soak them in a small bowl of water for 5 minutes, then toast in a moderately hot skillet until fragrant.

• All shelled nuts, but especially walnuts, have a rancid taste before they are roasted. Place walnuts in a saucepan, cover with cold water and bring to a vigorous boil for 5 minutes. Immediately drain into a sieve, spread on a baking sheet or toaster oven pan and roast in a 325 degree oven for 30 minutes, turning the nuts over after the first 15 minutes. When the nuts cool they will have an intense, nutty flavor without the bitter, rancid taste.

• If you use a full fat product such as olive oil or butter in a recipe, you can cut the fat in the recipe by using reduced fat versions of other ingredients. In this way, the dish will still have that mouth-satisfying taste of fat without all the calories.

• Purchase several sprayers for oils, such as Misto or Quickmist and use them to lightly coat cookware or ingredients with a film of oil when cooking. This will easily cut down on the amount of fat in any recipe.

• Start every meal, like the French, by nibbling on some protein first if you want to get glucagon levels rising as quickly as possible.

• If you are going to sear-roast a dish for dinner, start the oven as soon as you get into the kitchen, as it takes about 20 minutes for the oven to reach 500 degrees.

• Use colorful votive candle holders to serve melted butter or sauces. This will make any serving of fat look big for its size.

• Purchase two fajita pans from a restaurant supply store for sear-roasting. One should be cast iron for meat and the other steel or aluminum for fish. They will easily go from stovetop to oven for fast roasting without any oil.

• Select a wok that suits your stovetop. If you have a gas stove, purchase a round bottom wok and place it directly over the jets without the grill in place. For an electric stove, choose a flat-bottom wok so the coils are in direct contact with the bottom of the pan. Always cook with a wok on high heat.

• When stir-frying, always proceed to the next step when an ingredient changes color. In this way you will never overcook a dish.

• Always serve stir-fried food immediately. Danny

Kaye once prepared a Chinese dinner and shouted "don't look at it!" when he served it to me...and he meant it! Otherwise, the texture of the food will change as it steams on the plate.

• Purchase only fresh spices and herbs and throw out any that are over 6 months old if you want to enjoy the maximum fragrance and flavor they impart to a dish.

• Try to incorporate one new food each week into your diet.

• NEVER skip breakfast.

• Get over thinking of foods as "breakfast" foods, or "dinner" foods. Eat any food, any time.

• Select foods that have a glycemic index rating of 70 or less for the best results.

• Eat at least two fruits every day.

• If you don't want to destroy the healing compounds in garlic, peel the cloves and let them sit for 10 minutes so that oxygen can activate allinase, the protective enzyme that works as an antioxidant.

• Adding spices from the capsaicin family, such as chili peppers, paprika, hot sauces or chipotles, can stimulate your stomach to empty.

• Put vinaigrette dressings into a plastic hairdressing bottle and squeeze out the correct amount into a measuring spoon to be sure you're not "supersizing" your salad dressing.

sear-roasting fish, meat or fowl

An oven-proof skillet and two quick steps can give you food that is seared but still tender on the inside. It all starts by setting your oven to 500 degrees the moment you step into the kitchen. A standard oven will take about 20 minutes to achieve an internal temperature of 500 degrees, so take advantage of the time for preparation and setting the table.

For meat and poultry, I like to sear it first on the stove to get good color and flavor before putting the pan into the oven, where roasting completes the cooking without toughening the food. So here are

"The Rules"

• Be sure to bring the fish, poultry or meat to room temperature so that it will cook thoroughly.

• Be certain the food is thoroughly dry before you season it and put it into a hot pan or the moisture will interfere with the browning.

• Heat the skillet (or fajita pan) over a high flame until you can't hold your hand over it for longer than the count of 3.

• Don't let the oil smoke—it's bad for your health!

• Leave the food ALONE in the skillet. No poking or nudging. Use tongs so as not to pierce the food and let the juices escape.

• Use an oven thermometer to verify the oven has reached an internal temperature of 500 degrees.

• Flip the food over and immediately place the pan into the oven.

• Cook beef (6 ounces) 3 minutes for medium-rare; poultry for 4 minutes and fish for 3 minutes.

• If you prefer NOT to sear seafood, place the fish on a cold pan and roast for 10 minutes/per inch of thickness.

• Beware the handle of the pan when you remove it from the oven. It will be blazing hot!

Thanks to the Reynolds people, you can now purchase aluminum foil bags to cook "en papillote" anything you like—vegetables, fish, or chicken. It's all very simple. Just place the vegetables on the bottom of the bag, add the fish or poultry on top and seal the bag. Place it on a baking sheet in the oven at 450 degrees and bake for 20 minutes. All the juices remain in the bag and you have cooked your meal without any additional oil. To serve, just cut the bag open on the top, watching for any steam that may burn your hands.

Finally, never, never leave an oven thermometer inside when automatically cleaning an oven if you ever hope to read the temperature again.

It's so beautifully arranged on the plate—
you know someone's fingers
have been all over it.
~Julia Child~

chapter three

eggs

basil pistou omelette

classic french omelette

rogue river salmon omelette

french feta and zucchini frittata

allah's sunrise

basil pistou omelette

Pistou is the French version of Italian pesto, only the pine nuts are missing. Here I have used it to make a wonderful flavoring for a large omelette. Use only fresh basil leaves for the best flavor.

Serves 8
per portion
Calories: 94
Protein: 8 g
Carbs: 1 g
Fat: 6 g
Sat: 2 g

3 garlic cloves, chopped
1 cup fresh basil leaves, washed and dried
sea salt, white pepper
1 tablespoon extra-virgin olive oil
1/2 cup grated Parmesan cheese
4 eggs and 4 egg whites
1 tablespoon water

Put the garlic, basil, salt, pepper and 1 tablespoon oil in a food processor and blend until smooth. Add the cheese, a little at a time, until a very stiff paste forms. Set aside.

Whisk the eggs with salt, pepper and water until foamy. Spray a mist of olive oil on a large, nonstick omelette pan and heat until it is very hot. Add the egg mixture and let it cook 5 seconds. As the eggs begin to set, lift the edge with a fork and tilt the pan to run the eggs underneath. Continue until almost set but still slightly soft inside, about 30 seconds. Remove from the heat.

Quickly spread the pistou over the eggs and fold the omelette onto a serving plate to form a slight roll. Serve immediately.

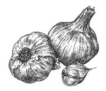

classic french omelette

Serves 2
per portion
Calories: 139
Protein: 16 g
Carbs: 7 g
Fat: 5 g
Sat: 1 g

The first thing I was taught at cooking school in France was how to make an omelette. I've adapted this recipe to include soy and my favorite herbs de Provence.

1 teaspoon extra-virgin olive oil
1/2 cup zucchini, diced
2 green onions, sliced
1 large egg and 3 egg whites
3 teaspoons soy powder
1/2 cup water
1/4 teaspoon herbs de Provence (see Resources)
sea salt

In a small nonstick skillet saute the zucchini and green onions over medium heat until soft.

In a separate bowl beat the eggs and egg white with the soy powder and add enough water for consistency. Pour the mixture over the vegetables and season with salt and herbs de Provence. Split the cherry tomatoes in half and place on the left side of the omelette. When the mixture is nearly set, slide the omelette onto a plate, tipping the pan to fold the omelette in half.

*Omelettes are never made
without breaking eggs.*
~Robespierre~

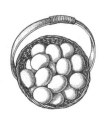

rogue river salmon omelette

Fishing on the Rogue River in Oregon is one of the simple delights in life. Chinook, Steelhead and Coho salmon run the river year round creating quite a boat traffic jam during high season. This delicious omelette is a fragrant reminder of the bounties of nature.

Serves 2
per portion
Calories: 186
Protein: 20 g
Carbs: 5 g
Fat: 9 g
Sat: 3 g

1 large egg and 3 egg whites
sea salt
pepper
3 ounces smoked salmon
1 ounce goat cheese
4 small cherry tomatoes, split in half
2 tablespoons fresh parsley

Preheat oven to 350 degrees. In a small electric mixing bowl, beat egg whites with salt and pepper till stiff peaks form. In another bowl, lightly beat yolks with a fork. Fold whites into yolks.

Lightly grease an oven proof nonstick skillet and place over medium-high heat. Spread the egg mixture in the pan. Cook 3 to 5 minutes or until the bottom is lightly golden.

Place skillet in the hot oven on a medium rack and bake for 3 minutes or until nearly dry.

Dot with the goat cheese, salmon, tomatoes and parsley and bake 1 minute more. To serve, fold the omelette in half.

Probably one of the most private things in the world is an egg until it is broken.
~M.F.K. Fisher~

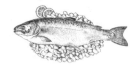

french feta and zucchini frittata

Serves 4
per portion
Calories: 175
Protein: 11 g
Carbs: 3 g
Fat: 13 g
Sat: 6 g

This is a rich dish, but well worth splurging some fat calories on for a special breakfast.

3 large eggs plus 4 egg whites
1/2 cup half-and-half
2 teaspoons extra-virgin olive oil
1 cup zucchini noodles (p. 91)
2 ounces fresh French feta cheese
1 teaspoon chopped dill

Preheat the broiler. In a a large bowl beat the eggs with the half-and-half and season lightly with salt and pepper.

In a heavy 9-inch oven-proof skillet, warm the olive oil over moderately high heat. When the oil begins to shimmer, add the eggs. Reduce the heat to moderately low and scatter the zucchini noodles over the eggs. Dot with the cheese and sprinkle with the dill. Cover and cook until almost set, about 12 minutes.

Broil the frittata for about 2 minutes or until the eggs are set. Cut into wedges and serve.

This recipe is certainly silly.
It says to separate eggs, but it doesn't say
how far to separate them.
~ Gracie Allen ~

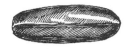

allah's sunrise

This recipe comes from the Middle East and can be made as spicy as you or your family can tolerate. I enjoyed it one morning as the sun was rising over the Great Atlas Mountains in Morocco. The owner of the little store on the route to Marrakech let me watch him prepare this regional dish while his goat nibbled on the few bunches of grass outside the door.

Serves 2
per portion
Calories: 197
Protein: 9 g
Carbs: 19 g
Fat: 10 g
Sat: 2.6 g

2 teaspoons extra virgin olive oil
1/3 cup chopped white onion
1/2 green bell pepper, seeded and cut into strips
1/2 poblano or red bell pepper,
    seeded and cut into strips
1 jalapeno pepper, raw, seeded and cut into tiny strips
    (retain the seeds and add for additional hotness)
8 ounces Muir Glen organic crushed tomatoes
    (see Resources)
2 teaspoons cayenne pepper or Aleppo pepper
    (see Resources)
sea salt
2 large eggs
Freshly ground black pepper to taste

Heat an empty cast iron skillet dry on medium heat, then add the olive oil and saute the onions and sweet peppers until soft, about 5 minutes, stirring with a wooden spoon.

Add the jalapeno and tomatoes and cook until the mixture just begins to thicken, about 8 minutes. Add the Aleppo or cayenne pepper and some sea salt to taste and adjust the seasoning for your preference.

Break one egg at a time into a bowl and slide it into the skillet while the tomato and pepper mixture is simmering. Cook for another 8 minutes, spooning the sauce over the eggs until they are set. Divide the dish in half and serve in individual bowls topped with black pepper.

chapter four
salads

chopped confetti tomato salad

crab with spicy orange dressing

cucumber-yogurt salad

grilled chicken and mandarin orange salad

lemon chicken

moroccan orange salad

shrimp salad

strawberries and feta salad

tuna and white bean salad

grilled steak and asparagus salad

apple, walnut, grapes and celery salad

chopped confetti tomato salad

When tomatoes are in season, I love to visit a local grower and get juicy red, yellow and orange tomatoes right off the vine. Any combination of tomatoes will work, but the colors add a festive touch to the table.

2 1/2 pounds yellow, orange and red tomatoes,
    cut into 1/2 inch pieces
1 small red onion, cut into 1/4 inch pieces
1/4 cup freshly squeezed lime juice
1/2 cup chopped fresh cilantro
sea salt
1 tablespoon extra-virgin olive oil
1 tablespoon whole coriander seeds

    Combine the tomatoes, onion, lime juice and cilantro in a bowl. Salt to taste and set aside.

    Heat the oil in a small skillet over medium-high heat until very hot. Add the coriander seeds; let fry until they pop, about 5 seconds. Immediately remove from heat, and pour the oil and seeds over the tomato salad. Stir gently to combine. Serve within 1 to 2 hours.

Serves 8
per portion
Calories: 52
Protein: 2 g
Carbs: 8 g
Fat: 2 g
Sat: <1 g

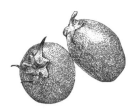

crab with spicy orange dressing

Serves 6
per portion
Calories: 138
Protein: 13 g
Carbs: 10 g
Fat: 5 g
Sat: 2 g

This dressing is excellent on shrimp, scallops or lobster and makes the fennel unusually sweet. Try using grapefruit juice instead of orange for another tasty variation. I have even served sections of grapefruit with this salad.

1 medium bulb fennel
1 tablespoon extra-virgin olive oil
3 tablespoons lemon juice
sea salt, pepper
2 cups fresh squeezed orange juice
     (grapefruit or lime)
1 teaspoon ancho chili powder (see Resources)
1 tablespoon unsalted butter
3 cans fancy white crab meat, picked for shells
1 1/2 tablespoons ground cumin
1/4 teaspoon cayenne pepper
8 basil leaves

Trim the top and bottom of the fennel bulb, then quarter lengthwise and slice the quarters into 1/8 inch slices. Place in a mixing bowl and toss with the olive oil, 2 tablespoons lemon juice and season to taste with salt and pepper.

In a small saucepan, bring the orange juice, remaining lemon juice and chili powder to a simmer over medium-high heat. Reduce to 1/3 cup, 15-17 minutes. Remove from the heat and whisk in the butter.

Drain the crab and check for any shell fragments. Mix with the ground cumin and cayenne pepper.

To serve, mound the fennel strips on the plate, press down in the middle and arrange the crab meat mixture on top. Drizzle the reduced orange dressing around the base of the fennel and over the crab.

Stack basil leaves and cut in julienne strips. Sprinkle on top of the crab.

cucumber-yogurt salad

This cooling salad has many names in the eastern and Mediterranean culture and even appears in Egypt and the Middle East. To make the best tasting salad, drain the yogurt for 2 hours before mixing.

2 cups whole milk yogurt
sea salt
1/2 medium cucumber, peeled and seeded
3 to 4 garlic cloves, mashed in a mortar and pestle
1 tablespoon chopped fresh dill
2 teaspoons fresh mint
2 teaspoons extra-virgin olive oil
1 tablespoon lemon juice

Serves 6
per portion
Calories: 70
Protein: 3 g
Carbs: 5 g
Fat: 4 g
Sat: 2 g

Combine the yogurt and 1/4 teaspoon sea salt in a cheesecloth-lined strainer over a bowl and let it drain for 2 hours.

Grate the cucumber with a coarse grater to make 1 cup total. Place the grated cucumber in another cheesecloth-lined strainer. Salt lightly and let drain 30 minutes.

Combine the yogurt, cucumber, garlic, herbs and olive oil. Mix well. Add the lemon juice to taste and season with salt. Let sit 1 hour before using.

Salad is not a meal.
It is a style.
~Fran Lebowitz~

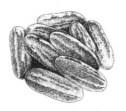

grilled chicken and mandarin orange salad

Serves 4
per portion
Calories: 273
Protein: 33 g
Carbs: 31 g
Fat: 4 g
Sat: 1 g

This salad is a frequent meal at my household and is so easy to make. Just serve with a glass of sparkling mineral water and voilá!

2 cans mandarin oranges
sea salt, pepper
1 cup fresh orange juice
1/2 cup rice wine vinegar
4 boneless, skinless chicken breasts (3 ounces each)
6 cups baby spinach leaves
1/2 small red onion, thinly sliced

In a bowl, combine the liquid from the mandarin oranges with the fresh orange juice and vinegar. Season with salt and pepper.

Split the dressing into two bowls.

Marinate the chicken breasts in one bowl of the dressing for 15 minutes. Grill the chicken until done, about 5 minutes per side.

Toss the spinach leaves with the remaining bowl of dressing and arrange on chilled individual serving plates. Cut each chicken breast crosswise into slices and arrange them along with the oranges on top of the spinach. Strew each salad with the red onions and serve immediately.

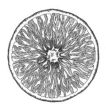

lemon chicken

This version of chicken is full of lemon flavor and bite. I use lemons preserved Morrocan style to add an exotic taste to this dish. Try freezing the chicken so it is easier to slice thinly.

1 1/4 pound skinless, boneless chicken breast halves,
    partially frozen
1 tablespoon canola oil
2 cups dry white wine
Juice of lemon
sea salt, pepper
1 bunch watercress, stems discarded
1 large head radicchio leaves, separated
2 preserved lemons,
    thinly sliced crosswise for garnish*

Serves 6
per portion
Calories: 170
Protein: 13 g
Carbs: 1 g
Fat: 3 g
Sat: <1 g

Using a sharp knife, thinly slice each chicken breast half on the diagonal 1/2 inch thick. Pound the chicken slices in a plastic bag until they are 1/4 inch thick.

Heat a large skillet on medium high heat dry, then add 1 tablespoon oil and half the chicken and cook until barely done, about 1 minutes per side; it will still be opaque in places. Transfer the chicken to a plate and repeat with the rest of the chicken, adding oil as necessary.

Carefully add the wine and lemon juice to the skillet, season with salt and pepper and bring to a boil over high heat. Return the chicken to the skillet and cook, stirring constantly, until the slices are white, about 2 to 3 minutes.

Line a platter with the watercress and radicchio and arrange the chicken slices on top. Garnish with the preserved lemon slices and serve immediately.

* To preserve lemons, rinse and scrub lemons or limes to remove any wax. Cut each fruit almost into four pieces by making cuts at right angles to each other from one end of the fruit almost to the other, leaving enough fruit uncut so that the lemon can be opened without falling apart, about 1/2

inch. Generously salt the exposed flesh with sea salt, using at least 3 tablespoons per pound of fruit. Put the salted fruits in a big, clean jar and cover with fresh lemon juice or water. Lemon juice gives a better flavor, but don't use bottled lemon juice. Put on the lid and leave the jar at room temperature for four or five weeks.

moroccan orange salad

Serves 4
per portion
Calories: 70
Protein: 1 g
Carbs: 10 g
Fat: 4 g
Sat: <1 g

This salad was served to me in Agadir, Morocco where the evening ocean breeze is filled with the fragrance of roses. You can make this salad with either daikon (a large white radish) or fennel. One taste and your guests will be looking for your magic lamp, so make plenty.

2 small oranges
1 daikon
mint springs

Dressing:
1 tablespoon lemon juice
2 teaspoons orange-flower water (see Resources)
1 tablespoon extra-virgin olive oil
sea salt, pepper
1 tablespoon chopped mint

Peel the oranges, removing the pith and slice. Peel the daikon and slice in thin circles. Arrange the daikon and oranges in an alternating pattern on a dish.

Make the dressing by whisking together lemon juice, orange-flower water, olive oil, salt and pepper. Pour dressing over the slices and sprinkle with the chopped mint and refrigerate.

Garnish with mint sprigs and serve.

shrimp salad

Here's an example of menomaise at work with shrimp.

1 pound extra-large shrimp, peeled and deveined
2 tablespoons lemon juice
sea salt, white pepper
One bag of romaine lettuce or 2 large heads
6 tablespoons menomaise (recipe on p. 128)

Serves 4
per portion
Calories: 183
Protein: 28 g
Carbs: 5 g
Fat: 6 g
Sat: 0 g

Marinate the shrimp in the lemon juice. Season with salt and pepper, then place under the broiler or on the grill, cooking them until uniformly pink and firm, about 2 minutes per side.

Assemble the salad in individual serving bowls. Tear the lettuce into pieces and toss with the menomaise.

Add the shrimp and serve.

strawberries and feta salad

An unusual but tasty way to serve strawberries and it's a snap to make. Try adding blueberries and grapes for another variation.

2 tablespoons orange juice, fresh squeezed
1 tablespoons white wine vinegar
2 teaspoons extra-virgin olive oil
2 bags (6 cups) salad greens
1 cup quartered strawberries
1/4 cup (1 ounce) crumbled French feta cheese

Serves 4
per portion
Calories: 60
Protein: 2 g
Carbs: 5 g
Fat: 4 g
Sat: 1 g

Combine first three ingredients in a small bowl and whisk together.

Place greens, strawberries and cheese in a large bowl and add orange juice mixture, tossing to coat.

tuna and white bean salad

Serves 4
per portion
Calories: 275
Protein: 31 g
Carbs: 24 g
Fat: 7 g
Sat: 1 g

This recipe can be found in almost any Italian trattoria. It's an example of fine, clean flavors—a specialty of Mediterranean cuisine.

Dressing:
3 tablespoons fresh lemon juice
1/2 teaspoon sea salt
1/4 teaspoon white pepper
1 teaspoon extra-virgin olive oil

Salad:
1 pound radicchio, leaves separated
One bag romaine lettuce or 2 large heads, torn
1 red bell pepper, quartered, stemmed and seeded
1 can tuna in oil (drain the oil and reserve for
     the dressing)
1 can (15 ounces) white cannellini beans, rinsed well
2 tablespoons fresh snipped chives
2 tablespoons fresh snipped dill
2 tablespoons Italian parsley, finely chopped
2 large shallots, coarsely chopped

In a small bowl, mix the lemon juice with the salt and pepper until dissolved. Drain the can of tuna and add the oil to the olive oil. Pour the oil in a steady stream while continuously whisking the lemon juice until emulsified.

Cut the radicchio leaves into strips and toss with the torn romaine leaves. Dice the bell pepper, then add all the remaining ingredients.

Toss the salad, then add the dressing to coat.

grilled steak and asparagus salad

This makes a wonderful, quick meal on a hot, summer day. Serve it with a garden-fresh salad for a meal even your friends will envy.

Vinaigrette:
1/4 cup hoisin sauce
1/4 cup white wine vinegar
1/4 cup canned fat free,
   reduced sodium chicken broth
4 teaspoons extra-virgin olive oil
4 teaspoons minced peeled fresh ginger
1 tablespoon soy sauce
2 teaspoons hot Chinese-style mustard
   or Dijon mustard

Salad:
1 tablespoon black peppercorns
2 teaspoons coriander seeds
2 teaspoons fennel seeds
1 1-pound top sirloin steak (about 1 inch thick)
Olive oil spray
1 pound thin asparagus spears, trimmed
3 medium-thin red onion slices
Orange slices

Serves 6
per portion
Calories: 162
Protein: 20 g
Carbs: 3 g
Fat: 8 g
Sat: 2 g

For vinaigrette: Blend all ingredients in a blender until smooth. Season with sea salt and pepper.

For salad: Grind peppercorns, coriander seeds and fennel seeds to a fine powder. Lightly spray steak with olive oil and sprinkle each side with salt, pepper and 1-1/2 teaspoons spice mix. Let stand 30 minutes.

Prepare barbecue (medium-high heat). Grill steak until cooked to desired doneness, about 5 minutes per side for medium-rare. Using tongs so as not to pierce the meat, transfer steak to a cutting board and let rest for 10 minutes, covered with foil.

While the steak is taking a much needed rest, (but not you!) spray the asparagus and onion slices with olive oil and sprinkle with salt and pepper. Grill asparagus until crisp-tender and slightly charred, turning often, about 5 minutes. Transfer to a plate and repeat with onion slices, keeping them intact.

Cut steak crosswise into thin slices. Arrange steak and asparagus on 6 plates. Drizzle with vinaigrette and garnish with onion rings and orange slices.

A woman is like a salad;
much depends on the dressing.
~Anonymous~

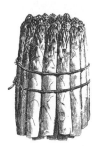

apple, walnut, grapes and celery salad

Poor Mr. Fawlty got a lesson in making a Waldorf salad when a rude, American guest stayed at his establishment. I promise you this salad will make no demands.

2 tablespoons reduced fat mayonnaise
1 tablespoon fresh lemon juice
1 crisp red apple
2 tablespoons walnuts
1/3 cup grapes
1-1/2 celery stalks
sea salt, pepper

Serves 2
per portion
Calories: 108
Protein: 1 g
Carbs: 16 g
Fat: 5 g
Sat: 1 g

In a non-metallic bowl, whisk together the mayonnaise and lemon juice, salt and pepper to taste until combined.

Cut celery and apple into 1-1/2-inch long thin julienne strips. Toss together the apple, walnuts, grapes and celery with the dressing.

There's somebody at every dinner party
who eats all the celery.
~Kin Hubbard~

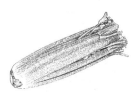

chapter five

soups

chayote soup with lemongrass and ginger

chilled cherry soup

chilled chick pea, tomato and yogurt soup

cream of bell pepper soup

cream of zucchini and anise soup

cucumber watercress soup

fennel and lemon soup

name your own vegetable soup

tomato and pumpkin soup

thai shrimp broth with lemongrass,
chili and ginger

chilled cantaloupe and mint soup

chayote soup with lemongrass and ginger

From a land of many islands comes a cuisine that mixes sweet and spicy tastes. Indonesians use tamarind, a sour tasting fruit from an evergreen tree that originated in Western Africa, instead of chayote. It is available in paste form in Asian and Latin markets. If you can't find fresh lemongrass, you can substitute 1/2 teaspoon lemon peel for each teaspoon of minced lemongrass. Kaffir lime leaves are fragrant and often sold frozen in Asian markets. You can substitute 1 tablespoon lime juice and 1/2 teaspoon grated lime peel for each lime leaf.

Serves 6
per portion
Calories: 38
Protein: 3 g
Carbs: 6 g
Fat: <1 g
Sat: 0 g

7 cups canned fat free, reduced sodium chicken broth
1 stalk fresh lemongrass, thinly sliced
    (about 2 teaspoons)
1 1-inch piece fresh ginger, sliced
3 fresh kaffir lime leaves
1/2 cinnamon Ceylon cinnamon stick (see Resources)
1/2 teaspoon ground nutmeg
1/4 teaspoon cayenne pepper
2 chayotes, peeled, rinsed, quartered, cored,
    thinly sliced crosswise
1/4 cup fresh lime juice
3/4 cup chopped fresh Italian parsley

Combine first 7 ingredients in a large pot and bring to a boil. Reduce heat and simmer 10 minutes to blend flavors. Strain liquid into bowl; return to same pot. Discard solids in strainer.

Bring liquid in pot to boil. Add chayotes; reduce heat and simmer until it is crisp-tender, about 7 minutes. Stir in lemon juice and parsley. Serve hot or chilled.

Soup is cuisine's kindest course.
~ Kitchen graffiti ~

chilled cherry soup

Serves 4
per portion
Calories: 122
Protein: 4 g
Carbs: 22 g
Fat: 3 g
Sat: 1 g

This is a great way to use soy in your diet with this refreshing, colorful soup. Save a few cherries to serve on top.

1 cup apple juice
1 cup pitted, fresh cherries
1 cup unsweetened soy milk
1 stick cinnamon, preferably Ceylon or Mexican

Combine all the ingredients except the cinnamon stick in the blender. Pour the mixture into a saucepan and bring to a simmer over low heat. Add the cinnamon stick and cook an additional 2 to 3 minutes, until thick. Remove the cinnamon stick and chill until cold.

*I have been on a constant diet
for the last two decades. By all accounts,
I should be hanging from a charm bracelet.*
~ Erma Bombeck ~

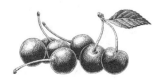

chilled chick pea, tomato and yogurt soup

Matthew Kenney of Mezze in New York serves this wonderful soup in the summer when the tomatoes are ripe and the afternoons long on sunshine. Chick peas are an ideal thickener for soup and they lose little of their nutty flavor when canned.

Serves 4
per portion
Calories: 225
Protein: 10 g
Carbs: 37 g
Fat: 5 g
Sat: 1 g

6 large, ripe tomatoes, peeled and seeded
2 teaspoons extra-virgin olive oil
2 cloves garlic, minced
1 teaspoon ground cardamom
1 teaspoon ground cumin
1 teaspoon ground ginger
2 cups canned chick peas, rinsed and drained
1 cup low-fat yogurt
sea salt, pepper
12 cilantro leaves, thinly sliced

Chop the tomatoes and set aside. Put the olive oil in a 4 quart saucepan over medium heat. Add the garlic and cook for 2 minutes, stirring to avoid burning. Add the tomatoes, cardamom, cumin and ginger and cook, uncovered for 15 minutes, or until the released tomato juices start to thicken.

Transfer the tomato-spice mixture to a food processor or blender and puree. Add the chick peas, 1/2 cup at a time, pulsing after each addition. The mixture should have a coarse texture. Pour into a bowl, stir in the yogurt and season with salt and pepper to taste. Refrigerate for at least 1 1/2 hours to overnight.

To serve, divide the soup among 4 chilled bowls and sprinkle with the cilantro.

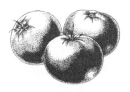

cream of bell pepper soup

Serves 4
per portion
Calories: 94
Protein: 3 g
Carbs: 7 g
Fat: 6 g
Sat: 2 g

With peppers coming in so many colors, you can make a rainbow of colored soups with this easy, quick recipe.

2 1/2 pounds single colored bell peppers
    (red, green, yellow, orange, purple)
2 teaspoons extra-virgin olive oil
1 cup chopped shallots
2 garlic cloves, minced
1 tablespoon chopped fresh thyme
3 cups or more canned vegetable broth
1/2 cup half and half
2 teaspoons red wine vinegar
1/2 teaspoon cayenne pepper
fresh basil, sliced or chiffonade

Char peppers over a gas flame or in a broiler until blackened on all sides. Enclose in a paper bag and let stand 10 minutes. Peel, seed and slice peppers.

Heat oil in a heavy large saucepan over medium heat. Add shallots, garlic and thyme and saute for 3 minutes. Add 3 cups of broth and all but 4 slices of roasted pepper. Simmer uncovered until peppers are very soft, about 20 minutes. Let cool 15 minutes.

Working in batches, puree the soup in a food processor until smooth. Return to the same pot and add half and half, vinegar and cayenne pepper. Rewarm the soup, thinning with additional broth as necessary and season with salt and pepper to taste. Garnish with a pepper strip and basil.

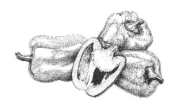

cream of zucchini and anise soup

This soup is delicious with any squash, including golden nugget or table queen. The fennel and anise-flavored Pernod complement the nutty taste of the squash. Float some edible flowers in the soup for an added effect.

Serves 4
per portion
Calories: 117
Protein: 3 g
Carbs: 13 g
Fat: 5 g
Sat: 2 g

2 teaspoons extra-virgin olive oil
6 cups chopped squash
    (zucchini, acorn, table queen or golden nugget)
1 large onion, chopped
2 cups water
4 garlic cloves, chopped
1-1/2 tablespoons fennel seeds
1 fresh thyme sprig
2 tablespoons whipping cream
2 tablespoons Pernod
sea salt, pepper
edible flowers

Heat olive oil in a large saucepan over medium heat. Add chopped squash and onion and saute until onion is translucent, about 15 minutes. Add 2 cups water, chopped garlic, 1-1/2 tablespoons fennel seeds and thyme sprig. Stir in 2 tablespoons whipping cream and Pernod. Simmer the soup uncovered 20 minutes. Remove the thyme sprig from the soup. Let cool 15 minutes.

Working in batches, puree the soup in a processor until smooth. Return to saucepan and heat before serving. Season with salt and pepper to taste. Ladle into bowls and top with an edible flower.

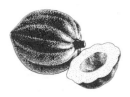

cucumber watercress soup

Serves 4
per portion
Calories: 119
Protein: 5 g
Carbs: 13 g
Fat: 6 g
Sat: 2 g

An English friend claimed this soup was prepared by her grandmother who lived in India during the days that country was considered "The Jewel" in Queen Victoria's crown. Just sipping this cool liquid out of a teacup will have you shouting "Long Live the Queen."

4 large cucumbers (3 1/2 pounds)
    peeled, seeded and cut into chunks
1 cup watercress sprigs
10 dill sprigs
2 tablespoons white wine vinegar
2 teaspoons extra-virgin olive oil
sea salt
1 1/2 cups whole milk yogurt
fresh pepper
4 radishes, finely chopped
2 scallions, finely chopped

In a blender puree the cucumbers, a handful at a time, until smooth. Add the watercress, half of the dill sprigs, vinegar, oil and 1 teaspoon of salt and puree until smooth.

Transfer the soup to a bowl and stir in the yogurt. Refrigerate until chilled, about 2 hours. Season with salt and pepper and pour into bowls. Garnish with the radishes, scallions and the remaining 4 sprigs of dill.

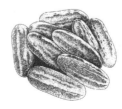

fennel and lemon soup

I am always looking for ways to serve unusual vegetables, and this one for fennel is easy, fast and delicious. It can be served either hot or chilled. Save some of the fennel leaves for garnish.

1 teaspoon extra-virgin olive oil
1 white onion, chopped
2 fennel bulbs, thinly sliced
2 1/2 cups chicken stock
1 cup milk 2%
sea salt, pepper
1 lemon, zested and juiced

Serves 4
per portion
Calories: 75
Protein: 4 g
Carbs: 10 g
Fat: 2 g
Sat: 1 g

Heat the skillet dry on high heat, then add the olive oil. Immediately reduce heat and add the onions. Cook over low heat for 5 minutes or until soft. Stir in the fennel pieces.

Add the stock and lemon zest and bring to a boil. Reduce the heat, cover and simmer for 20 minutes or until fennel is tender.

Transfer to a food processor and process until smooth. Add enough milk to give the desired consistency and season with salt and pepper. Stir in the lemon juice just before serving and garnish with some fennel leaves.

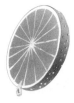

name your own vegetable soup

Serves 8
per portion
Calories: 87
Protein: 8 g
Carbs: 10 g
Fat: 3 g
Sat: 0 g

Asparagus is plentiful on the California coast and when it's in season I make use of every part. This soup can be turned into whatever you wish merely by using two pounds of fresh something.

2 cups fat free, reduced sodium chicken stock
3 cups water
1 pound yellow onions, chopped
3 cloves garlic, coarsely chopped
1 teaspoon extra-virgin olive oil
2 pounds fresh *something*
    (either asparagus, spinach, broccoli)
6 oz tofu
sea salt, white pepper
2 tablespoons fresh tarragon, minced

Place the stock and water into a large pot and bring to a boil.

Heat a skillet dry on high heat, then add the oil and saute the onions and garlic over medium heat until soft. Add the broccoli and season with the salt and pepper. Continue to saute the broccoli until it is bright green and starting to soften. Do not burn the onions and garlic.

Empty the vegetable mixture into the boiling stockpot and cover. Return to a boil then uncover and boil for 5 to 10 minutes, being sure not to make the broccoli lose its color.

Remove from the heat, add the tofu and puree. Add the tarragon and serve after correcting the seasoning.

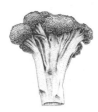

tomato and pumpkin soup

My grandmother was a Canadian wheat farmer's wife and she often served soup for breakfast. This unique take on a winter soup will have you in a "field of dreams" before you know it.

2 cups white onions, chopped
1 teaspoon canola oil
1/2 teaspoon nutmeg
1 can (14 1/2 oz.) pumpkin (not the one for pie)
1 can (14 1/2 oz.) Muir Glen organic tomatoes, chopped
1/4 cup finely chopped parsley
4 cups fat free, reduced sodium chicken stock
1 cup non-fat yogurt
6 oz tofu
sea salt, pepper to taste

Serves 8
per portion
Calories: 110
Protein: 8 g
Carbs: 14 g
Fat: 3 g
Sat: 0 g

Heat the skillet dry on high heat, then add the oil and saute the onions on medium heat until limp and translucent.

Add nutmeg, pumpkin, tomatoes, parsley and chicken stock and simmer for 5 minutes.

Add the yogurt and tofu, puree and season to taste.

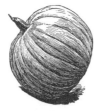

thai shrimp broth with lemongrass, chili and ginger

Serves 4
per portion
Calories: 121
Protein: 20 g
Carbs: 2 g
Fat: 3 g
Sat: 1 g

I often frequent the numerous Thai restaurants in my area and enjoy a bowlful of this heavenly soup whenever I can. Just don a cooley hat and imagine yourself floating on a sampan in Bangkok Harbor.

1/2 pound uncooked, large shrimp
4 14-1/2-ounce cans fat free, reduced sodium
  chicken broth
8 thin slices fresh lemongrass
2 tablespoons finely chopped ginger
1 tablespoon minced garlic
1 tablespoon finely chopped fresh basil
1 tablespoon finely chopped fresh mint
1 tablespoon finely chopped cilantro
1 small serrano chili, stemmed,
  thinly sliced into rounds
1 teaspoon fresh lime juice
4 thin lime slices

Peel and devein shrimp; reserve shells. Halve shrimp lengthwise and transfer to a small bowl. Cover and chill.

Combine reserved shrimp shells, broth and next 4 ingredients in a large pot. Bring to a boil. Reduce heat; simmer uncovered 20 minutes to blend flavors, stirring and skimming surface occasionally.

Strain broth into a large bowl, pressing on the solids with the back of a spoon to release as much liquid as possible; discard solids. Return broth to the pot. Bring to a simmer. Remove the heat and add the shrimp, herbs, chili and lime juice. Cover and let stand until shrimp are opaque, stirring once, about 2 minutes.

Ladle into bowls. Garnish with lime wedges.

chilled cantaloupe and mint soup

This soup is wonderful in the summertime when melons are in abundance. Try using spearmint instead of peppermint for a unique flavor. If you want to get fancy, make another version with honeydew melons and pour the two into the same dish side by side for a real treat.

1 medium cantaloupe
1 1/2 tablespoons fresh mint
1 cup yogurt, low fat
1/2 cup dry white wine

Puree the cantaloupe and mint in a blender.
Pour into a bowl and mix with the yogurt and wine.
Chill overnight.

Serves 4
per portion
Calories: 104
Protein: 4 g
Carbs: 15 g
Fat: 1 g
Sat: 0 g

"How long does getting thin take?"
Pooh asked anxiously.
~ A.A.Milne ~

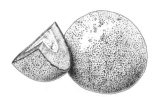

chapter six

seafood

orange roughy with orange, caper and olive sauce

ginger shrimp in napa cabbage

halibut with artichokes, zucchini and tomatoes

mussels in chipotle chili broth

provencal style lemon sole

shrimp with two mushrooms

sea bass with chili and saffron

seared black scallops

smoked salmon with apples

tu tu tun lodge grilled salmon

baked basque cod

sear-roasted halibut

orange roughy with orange, caper and olive sauce

This fish has a wonderful texture when baked with this sauce. By using a very hot oven, the fish remains moist and flaky.

1 orange
1/2 cup finely chopped seeded plum tomatoes
1/4 cup fresh orange juice
3 tablespoons minced red onion
1-1/2 tablespoons fresh lemon juice
2 teaspoons extra-virgin olive oil
5 minced Kalamata olives
1 tablespoon chopped, drained capers
1 teaspoon chopped fresh rosemary
4 3-ounce orange roughy fillets

Serves 4
per portion
Calories: 190
Protein: 14 g
Carbs: 13 g
Fat: 9 g
Sat: <1 g

Preheat oven to 500 degrees. Remove peel and white pith from orange. Cut twenty 2-inch-long, 1/8-inch wide strips of orange peel and reserve. Chop orange; place in a small, non-metallic bowl. Add tomatoes, onion, lemon juice, olive oil, olives, capers and rosemary to the chopped orange; stir to blend. Season with salt and pepper to taste.

Spray a glass baking dish with olive oil and arrange the fish in it. Sprinkle orange strips evenly over fish. Season with salt and pepper.

Bake until fish is opaque in center, about 10 minutes.

Spoon sauce over fish and serve.

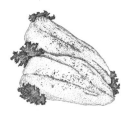

ginger shrimp in napa cabbage

Makes 12 wraps
per wrap
Calories: 54
Protein: 12 g
Carbs: 1 g
Fat: 1 g
Sat: <1 g

This recipe demonstrates how useful cabbage leaves can be as a wrap for shrimp, beef or chicken dishes. Like grape leaves, they are low in calories yet high in fiber.

One unpeeled 4-inch piece of fresh ginger
1 teaspoon sea salt
4 cups water
24 medium shrimp, peeled and deveined
12 Napa cabbage leaves,
    halved lengthwise, ribs removed
2 teaspoons Asian black bean sauce
1/2 cup radish sprouts

In a food processor, finely chop the ginger. Transfer to a saucepan, add the salt and water and bring to a boil. Simmer over moderate heat for 10 minutes. Strain the ginger broth through a fine sieve, discarding the ginger. Return the broth to the pan and bring to a boil. Add the shrimp and cook over high heat until just opaque, about 1 minute. Remove the shrimp to a plate with a slotted spoon and let cool. Let the cooking liquid cool too, then add the shrimp and refrigerate until chilled, at least 30 minutes. Drain the shrimp and pat dry.

In a large pot of boiling water, cook the cabbage until tender, about 2 minutes. Drain and let cool under running water, then dry the cabbage leaves thoroughly with paper towels.

Cut the cabbage into 6-by-1-inch strips. Set a shrimp at one end of a cabbage strip, top with a scant teaspoon of the black bean sauce and a few of the sprouts and roll up the shrimp in the cabbage strip. Repeat with the remaining ingredients.

There is no love sincerer than the love of food.
~ George Bernard Shaw ~

halibut with artichokes, zucchini and tomatoes

This dish is quick and simple. Try using sea bass or orange roughy if halibut is not fresh.

1 6-ounce jar marinated artichoke hearts
2 3-ounce halibut fillets
8 ounces plum tomatoes, chopped
1 zucchini, cut into rounds
3 tablespoons chopped, fresh basil
2 garlic cloves, minced
3/4 bottle clam juice

Preheat oven to 475 degrees. Drain marinade from artichokes into a 9-inch diameter glass pie dish. Add fish; turn to coat with marinade. Sprinkle fish with salt and pepper. Scatter artichokes, tomatoes, zucchini, basil and garlic around fish. Pour clam juice over the fish and bake until fish is just opaque in the center, about 20 minutes.

Serves 2
per portion
Calories: 208
Protein: 27 g
Carbs: 18 g
Fat: 3 g
Sat: <1 g

The artichoke is a trick vegetable.
~ Groucho Marx ~

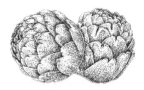

mussels in chipotle chili broth

Serves 4
per portion
Calories: 178
Protein: 15 g
Carbs: 11 g
Fat: 5 g
Sat: 1 g

One year, for my birthday, friends took me to three restaurants in one night, where we ate mussels prepared in different styles. This recipe, from Rocking Horse Café Mexicano, is a great way to serve the new, farm raised mussels. Do like the natives and use the shell to scoop up the spicy broth before sucking the mussels right off. ¡Ay Caramba!

2 teaspoons peanut oil
3 garlic cloves, minced
1 tablespoon minced canned chipotle chilis
3 pounds mussels, (12 ounces meat only)
    scrubbed and debearded*
1/2 cup dry white wine
1 cup fish stock or bottled clam juice
6 plum tomatoes, coarsely chopped
5 Kalamata olives, pitted and sliced
4 tablespoons chopped fresh cilantro
sea salt to taste

Heat a large, heavy pot over medium-high heat and add oil. Add garlic and saute for 30 seconds (do not burn the garlic). Mix in the chipotle chilis, then add the wine, mussels and stock; cover and cook 4 minutes. Mix in tomatoes, olives and 2 tbsp. cilantro. Cover and cook until mussels open, about 3 minutes longer. Discard any mussels that don't open, then season to taste with sea salt.

Transfer mussels and broth to individual bowls and sprinkle with the remaining 2 tbsp. of cilantro.

* To check if your mussels are alive, put them in the freezer for 5 minutes. Any mussels that remain open should be discarded.

provencal style lemon sole

This dish is quick to make and works equally well with halibut or even scallops if you are unable to find fresh lemon sole.

2 navel oranges
2 teaspoons extra-virgin olive oil
1 large red onion, thinly sliced
1 tablespoon thinly sliced garlic
3/4 cup (6 ounces) canned tomatoes, chopped
3/4 cup dry white wine
5 Kalamata olives, pitted and cut into thin slivers
4 4-ounce lemon sole fillets
Chives, cut into 1 1/2-inch lengths for garnish

Serves 4
per portion
Calories: 210
Protein: 23 g
Carbs: 13 g
Fat: 4 g
Sat: 1 g

Using a sharp knife, peel the oranges, removing all of the white pith and cut between the membranes to release the orange sections into a medium bowl.

Heat the oil in a large, deep skillet. Add the onion and garlic and cook over moderate heat until lightly browned, about 5 minutes. Stir in the tomatoes and wine and season with salt and pepper. Cook until the liquid is slightly reduced, about 4 minutes. Add the olives and set the fish fillets on top in a single layer. Season with salt and pepper, cover and cook until the fillets easily flake, about 7 minutes. Carefully transfer the fish to a platter.

Stir the oranges into the sauce and spoon the sauce onto plates. Set the fillets on top. Garnish with the chives and serve at once.

An onion can make people cry,
but there's no vegetable
that can make them laugh.
~Anonymous~

shrimp with two mushrooms

Serves 4
per portion
Calories: 165
Protein: 24 g
Carbs: 7 g
Fat: 5 g
Sat: 1 g

While visiting the island of Santorini, I tasted this wonderful dish made with two mushrooms and freshly caught shrimp. The smell of the salt air still lingers in my mind whenever I make this.

1/2 cup dried porcini mushrooms (about 1/2 ounce)
1/2 cup dried morel mushrooms (about 1/2 ounce)
2 cups hot water
2 teaspoons extra-virgin olive oil
1 pound large, uncooked, cleaned shrimp
1/3 cup Madeira
2 tablespoons chopped fresh Italian parsley
2 teaspoons sesame seeds

Place dried mushrooms in a bowl and cover with the hot water. Let stand for 30 minutes, or until soft. Using a slotted spoon, transfer the mushrooms to a small bowl, reserving the soaking liquid.

Heat a large, nonstick pan over moderate heat and add the olive oil. Add mushrooms and saute 2 minutes. Add shrimp; saute 1 minute. Add the wine and simmer until almost all the liquid evaporates, about 1 minute. Add 1/3 cup reserved mushroom soaking liquid (leave the sediment behind). Saute until shrimp are just cooked through, about 2 minutes.

Mix in the parsley and divide among 4 plates. Sprinkle with the sesame seeds.

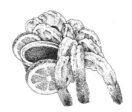

sea bass with chili and saffron

Sea bass is a popular white fish with excellent texture. It takes on new flavors when treated with this Near East recipe.

2 red bell peppers
8 Italian tomatoes, peeled*
5 tablespoons chopped cilantro
2 cloves garlic, chopped
1/2 teaspoon ground cumin
1/2 teaspoon ancho chili powder
1/4 teaspoon saffron threads
1 teaspoon paprika
sea salt, pepper
pinch of cayenne
2 teaspoons spicy olive oil
4 fillets of sea bass, 4 ounces each
1/2 cup clam juice or fish stock
1 cup chick peas, rinsed and drained
harissa (optional—see Resources)

Serves 4
per portion
Calories: 261
Protein: 27 g
Carbs: 22 g
Fat: 7 g
Sat: 1 g

    Char the peppers on the stove over a hot flame. If you have an electric cooktop, then preheat the broiler and put the peppers on a sheet pan lined with foil and broil for about 15 minutes, turning once or twice to ensure they blister and blacken. Place in a paper bag and let cool. Peel, seed and cut into 1/2 inch wide strips. Set aside. Cut the tomatoes lengthwise and into eighths. Set aside.
    Preheat the oven to 350 degrees.
    In a small bowl, combine 2 tablespoons of the cilantro, garlic, cumin, chilis, saffron, paprika, salt, black pepper, cayenne and olive oil. If you wish a truly spicy version, add a dab of harissa. Rub each fillet with the mixture and add the remainder to the stock. Warm the stock in a small saucepan.
    Place the fish tightly in a baking dish. Spread the chick peas, tomatoes, and peppers evenly on top of the fish. Pour the stock over and cover with foil. Bake

for 15 minutes, remove the foil and bake 5 more minutes. Transfer the fish to a platter, surround with the vegetables and pour the cooking liquid over the fish. Sprinkle with the remaining cilantro.

To peel tomatoes, drop them in boiling water for 30 seconds, then drop in ice water. The peel will slip right off.

seared black scallops

Serves 2
per portion
Calories: 138
Protein: 12 g
Carbs: 9 g
Fat: 5 g
Sat: 1 g

I use the black seeds, called Nigella, common to Morocco and India. It gives a wonderful color contrast to the white scallops and imparts a sweet taste.

3 tablespoons Nigella or black seeds (see Resources)
1 1/2 teaspoon sea salt
1/8 teaspoon freshly ground black pepper
6 large sea scallops (about 5 ounces)
2 teaspoons extra-virgin olive oil

In a small bowl stir together the seeds, salt and pepper. Trim the scallops of any tough muscle that is attached on the side and pat scallops dry. Dip flat sides of each scallop in the seed mixture.

In a 12-inch nonstick skillet heat oil over moderately high heat until hot but not smoking and saute scallops on the flat sides until the seeds are fragrant and scallops are just cooked through, about 4 minutes total.

*I'd like to come back as an oyster.
Then I'd only have to be good
from September until April.*
~Gracie Allen~

smoked salmon with apples

This is another delicious way to serve salmon. The taste of apple cider compliments the sweetness of the apples and the peppery taste of watercress.

Serves 4
per portion
Calories: 237
Protein: 24 g
Carbs: 8 g
Fat: 12 g
Sat: 3 g

1 cup applewood hardwood chips
4 4-ounce salmon fillets seasoned with sea salt,
    white pepper
1/4 cup apple cider
3 teaspoons unsalted butter
1/2 teaspoon Dijon mustard
1/2 Granny Smith apple, cut into 4 pieces
1/2 julienned Red Delicious apple
1/2 teaspoon lemon juice
7 ounces watercress sprigs
1 large garlic clove, minced
1/4 cup radish sprouts

Soak the wood chips in warm water for 20 minutes, then drain. Light a small charcoal fire and when ready, add the chips and heat until smoking. Do not use lighter fluid as it will give a bitter taste to the fish.

Set the seasoned salmon on the rack and cover and smoke for about 20 minutes or until fragrant and cooked through. Transfer to a plate.

Heat 1/4 cup apple cider in a saucepan to boil. Over low heat add 2 teaspoons butter and mustard until incorporated. Adjust seasoning.

Cut the Granny Smith apple into wedges and julienne the Red Delicious apple and add to the bowl. Toss with lemon juice.

Melt the remaining 1 teaspoon of butter in a skillet and add the watercress and garlic and cook over high heat, tossing, until wilted, about 4 minutes. Season with salt and pepper and transfer to 4 shallow soup plates.

Arrange the salmon on the watercress and scatter the julienned apples around and garnish with the radish sprouts. Whisk the apple broth over high heat until foamy, then pour it around the salmon and serve.

tu tu tun lodge grilled salmon

*Serves 12
per portion
Calories: 250
Protein: 32 g
Carbs: <1 g
Fat: 12 g
Sat: 2 g*

As a neighbor of Dirk and Laurie van Zantes, owners of the Tu Tu Tun Lodge, I look forward to the day whole, fresh caught Rogue River salmon are served. Laurie uses fresh applewood from their orchard, but wood chips work nicely as well. It's worth buying a whole salmon, so invite lots of friends to share in this wonderful feast.

1 teaspoon extra-virgin olive oil
3 1/2 - 4 pound salmon fillet with the skin
1/4 cup dry white wine
2 teaspoons fresh lemon juice
2 teaspoons minced fresh garlic
1 tablespoon finely chopped fresh parsley
2 teaspoons fresh thyme leaves
sea salt, pepper to taste

Prepare a grill by opening vents and filling a chimney starter with charcoal and light. (Do not use lighter fluid). Charcoal will be ready when it is lightly coated with gray ash, 15 to 20 minutes. Mound lighted charcoal on opposite sides of grill bottom, leaving the middle clear. Spread apple branches that have been soaked in water overnight over the charcoal and position the rack. When wood begins to smoke, in about 2 minutes, grill is ready.

While the charcoal is lighting, use heavy duty foil in 2 layers and make a shallow baking pan just large enough to fit the salmon and put the pan on a large baking sheet to stabilize it. Spray foil with oil and put the salmon, skin side down, on foil. Pour wine and lemon juice evenly over the salmon and spray a small amount of oil over the fish. Sprinkle garlic, parsley, thyme, salt and pepper over the fish and carefully slide the foil package onto the center of the grill and cover. Grill salmon over indirect heat, without turning, until just cooked through, about 25 to 30 minutes.

baked basque cod

Cod is a simple fish widely available in the Basque region of Spain and is a mainstay in their cooking. Try making a mixture of vegetables available in the fresh produce section for a different variation. This also works well with red snapper.

Serves 4
per portion
Calories: 140
Protein: 21 g
Carbs: 6 g
Fat: 3 g
Sat: 1 g

2 teaspoons extra-virgin olive oil
1 green pepper, diced
1 white onion, finely chopped
2 tomatoes, peeled and diced
1 garlic clove, crushed
2 teaspoons fresh basil
4 cod fillets, skinned, approximately 4 ounces each
Juice of 1/2 lemon
sea salt, pepper
lemon slices for garnish

Heat oven to 375 degrees. Brush four large squares of foil with a little oil.

Mix together the bell pepper, onion, tomatoes, garlic and basil. Put a fillet in the center of each foil piece and top with the mixture.

Drizzle with lemon juice and the remaining oil and season with salt and pepper. Fold the foil into parcels and place on a baking sheet in the oven for 20 minutes or until the fish flakes easily.

Unwrap the foil and transfer the fish, vegetables and cooking juices onto serving plates.

Garnish with lemon slices and serve.

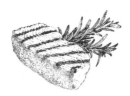

sear-roasted halibut

Serves 2
per portion
Calories: 183
Protein: 35 g
Carbs: 0 g
Fat: 4 g
Sat: <1 g

12 ounces fresh halibut fillet, about 1 inch thick
sea salt or seasoning of your choice

Heat the oven to 500 degrees for 20 minutes. Heat the roasting pan dry on high heat until you can't hold your hand over the pan for longer than the count of 3. Season the halibut with sea salt on both sides or with a seasoning mixture of your choice. Spray the roasting pan with olive oil and place the halibut on the pan to sear one side. This will take about 1 minute. Turn the halibut over and immediately place the pan in the oven and roast for 8 minutes.

There is nothing like good food,
good wine and a bad girl.
~Fortune Cookie~

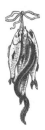

chapter seven

poultry

calcutta chicken in spinach
and yogurt sauce

chicken, tofu and watercress stir-fry

roasted turkey breast

chicken with spiced yogurt marinade

grilled chicken in cilantro-mint rub

indian turkey cutlets

lemon tarragon chicken

chicken breasts with thyme-lemon marinade

calcutta chicken in spinach and yogurt sauce

This dish is made with seasoning characteristic of the west Bengal region of India. For a truly authentic taste, use mustard oil instead of canola. Make sure you heat the mustard oil to the smoking point and let it smoke for 3 to 5 seconds before adding the ingredients. This tempers its pungency.

Serves 4
per portion
Calories: 235
Protein: 29 g
Carbs: 10 g
Fat: 8 g
Sat: 2 g

12 ounces boneless, skinless chicken breasts
1 bunch baby spinach leaves
1 medium white onion
4 large garlic cloves
1 small serrano chili
1 1-inch piece fresh gingerroot
1/2 teaspoon brown or black mustard seeds
1 tablespoon mustard oil or canola oil
2 teaspoons ground coriander seeds
1 cup plain, whole milk yogurt
1 teaspoon sea salt

Chop the chicken breasts into pieces. Discard the stems from the baby spinach leaves and chop enough spinach to measure 2 cups. Chop the onion and mince the garlic and the chili pepper. Peel the gingerroot and mince. With a spice grinder, coarsely grind the mustard seeds.

In a heavy 12-inch skillet, heat the mustard oil over high heat until smoking, then reduce the heat to moderate and cook the onion, garlic, serrano, gingerroot and mustard seeds, stirring until the onion begins to brown. Add the coriander and cook, stirring, 1 minute. Stir in the spinach and cook until it begins to wilt, about 30 seconds. Gradually add yogurt, stirring until well combined. Stir in the chicken pieces, salt and simmer the mixture until the chicken is cooked, about 5 minutes.

chicken, tofu and watercress stir-fry

Serves 6
per portion
Calories: 159
Protein: 26 g
Carbs: 1 g
Fat: 5 g
Sat: 1 g

Another fast, easy way to incorporate soy into your diet. Remember to let the wok heat up until you can't hold your hand over the pan longer than 3 seconds. Just add the oil and you'll be wokking the fat out of your diet.

1 teaspoon peanut oil
12 ounces boneless, skinless chicken breast,
    cut into strips
3 ounces firm tofu, cut into 1/2-inch cubes
4 tablespoons Chinese oyster sauce
1 cup water or fat free, reduced sodium chicken broth
4 cups watercress, cut into 2-inch lengths

Heat the pan over high heat dry, then add peanut oil and immediately add the chicken pieces and tofu cubes, stirring often to brown all sides. Combine the oyster sauce with the water or broth and stir the liquid into the stir-fry. Once it is hot, add the watercress and reduce the heat to low. Cover the pan and cook for one minute or until the chicken is cooked through and the watercress has wilted.

roasted turkey breast

per portion
3 ounces
Calories: 47
Protein: 10 g
Carbs: 0 g
Fat: <1 g
Sat: 0 g

This is so simple and delicious, you'll be wishing it was Thanksgiving every day.

1 turkey breast
California BBQ seasoning (p. 111)

Heat the oven to 350 degrees.
Take the turkey breast and season under the skin with the California BBQ seasoning. Place it in an oven-proof pan and roast for one hour.

chicken with spiced yogurt marinade

This dish is popular in Afghanistan where it works equally well with lamb and chicken. The perfume of saffron contrasts nicely with the piquancy of lemon juice and garlic in this tangy marinade. Don't use boneless chicken as it will not remain juicy on the grill.

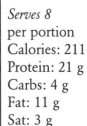

Serves 8
per portion
Calories: 211
Protein: 21 g
Carbs: 4 g
Fat: 11 g
Sat: 3 g

2 cups whole milk yogurt
2 tablespoons fresh lemon juice
4 garlic cloves, minced
1 medium yellow onion, minced
2 teaspoons ground coriander
1 teaspoon ground cumin
2 teaspoons sea salt
1 teaspoon white pepper
1/2 teaspoon saffron threads, crumbled
1/2 teaspoon cinnamon
8 chicken breasts and thighs, bone in, including skin

In a bowl combine the yogurt, lemon juice, garlic, onion, coriander, cumin, salt, pepper, saffron and cinnamon. Stir well to blend.

Place the chicken pieces in a large glass or ceramic dish and pour the marinade on top. Let marinate 4 hours or overnight.

Light a grill and cook the chicken pieces over a medium-hot fire, turning often, until lightly charred on both sides and just cooked through, about 10 minutes per side.

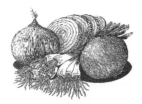

grilled chicken in cilantro-mint rub

Serves 8
per portion
Calories: 145
Protein: 25 g
Carbs: 3 g
Fat: 3 g
Sat: 1 g

This rub is excellent on pork or lamb but don't let it cook too long or the rub will darken. Serve with additional sauce on the side.

2 cups packed fresh flat-leaf parsley
2 cups cilantro
1 cup spearmint leaves
3 small cloves garlic, minced
1 small jalapeno, seeds and ribs removed,
    roughly chopped
1/4 cup plus 2 tablespoons fresh lemon juice
1 1/2 teaspoons sea salt
1/2 teaspoons ground cumin
8 skinless, boneless chicken breasts

Combine everything but the chicken in a food processor and blend until a thick paste forms. Remove half of the mixture and add 2 tablespoons water to make a sauce.

Place the paste in a plastic bag and add the chicken breasts, massaging the paste into each breast.

Heat an oil sprayed grill over medium high heat until very hot. Season the chicken with salt and pepper and cook the meat until done, about 4 minutes per side.

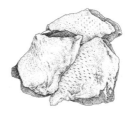

indian turkey cutlets

This is a great way to use those turkey slices in the meat department. Be careful not to soak them in the yogurt or they will take on a mealy characteristic.

2 large limes
1/3 cup plain low-fat yogurt
2 teaspoons canola oil
2 teaspoons minced, peeled gingerroot
1 teaspoon ground cumin
1 teaspoon ground coriander
sea salt
1 garlic clove, crushed with garlic press
1 1/2 pounds turkey cutlets
cilantro sprigs for garnish

Serves 6
per portion
Calories: 153
Protein: 28 g
Carbs: 3 g
Fat: 3 g
Sat: 1 g

From 1 lime, grate 1 teaspoon peel and squeeze 1 tablespoon juice. Cut the remaining lime into wedges; reserve wedges for squeezing juice over cooked cutlets. In large bowl, mix lime peel, lime juice, yogurt, canola oil, gingerroot, cumin, coriander, salt, and garlic until blended.

Just before grilling, add turkey cutlets to bowl with yogurt mixture, stirring to coat cutlets.

Place turkey cutlets on grill over medium heat. Cook cutlets 5 to 7 minutes until they just lose their pink color throughout. Serve with lime wedges. Garnish with cilantro sprigs.

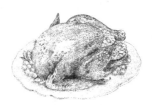

lemon tarragon chicken

Serves 4
per portion
Calories: 149
Protein: 24 g
Carbs: 0 g
Fat: 5 g
Sat: 1 g

A simple, classic French dish that takes so little time, but makes a great impression.

2 medium-size lemons
1 tablespoon chopped fresh tarragon
   or 1/2 teaspoon dried
2 teaspoons olive oil
sea salt, pepper
1 garlic clove, minced
4 small skinless, boneless chicken breasts,
   3 ounces each

From 1 lemon, grate enough peel to equal 2 teaspoons. Thinly slice half of second lemon; reserve slices for garnish. Squeeze juice from remaining 3 lemon halves into small bowl. Stir in lemon peel, tarragon, olive oil, salt, pepper, and garlic.

Toss chicken breast halves with the lemonjuice mixture. Heat skillet dry over high heat.

Place chicken breast halves in hot skillet; cook 5 minutes, brushing with remaining lemon-juice mixture in bowl. Turn chicken over and cook 5 minutes longer until juices run clear when thickest part of chicken breast is pierced with a knife. Garnish with lemon slices.

Let food be your medicine
and medicine your food.
~Hippocrates~

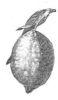

chicken breasts with thyme-lemon marinade

This dish is a regular at my house. It's quick, easy and very low in fat and calories. Serve it with steamed, fresh broccoli studded with toasted almonds for a real treat!

4 3-ounce boneless, skinless chicken breasts
3 tablespoons fresh lemon juice
1 tablespoon chopped fresh thyme
    or 1 teaspoon dried
2 teaspoons grated lemon peel
2 garlic cloves, pressed

Serves 4
per portion
Calories: 132
Protein: 24 g
Carbs: 1 g
Fat: 3 g
Sat: 1 g

Place chicken breasts in a plastic bag.

Mix the lemon juice, thyme, lemon peel and garlic in small bowl.

Pour the mixture over the chicken and massage the bag to cover all the chicken. Refrigerate one hour or up to one day.

Remove the chicken from the bag and grill for 3 minutes per side.

*Cuisine is when things
taste like themselves.
~ Curnonsky ~*

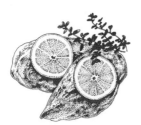

chapter eight

meat

filet mignon with castello blue cheese

flank steak in adobo seasoning

grilled leg of lamb with rosemary and garlic

moorish spicy lamb kebabs

pork chops with chipotle marinade

roast pork loin with garlic and rosemary

spicy beef with basil

cuban grilled skirt steak

filet mignon with castello blue cheese

This is one of my favorite ways to top a great filet. Just put a dab of this Danish triple cream blue cheese on a hot, grilled filet and watch it melt away your day. I roast the filet after searing on a hot griddle to insure the meat remains moist as it cooks.

Serves 1
per portion
Calories: 181
Protein: 19 g
Carbs: 0 g
Fat: 12 g
Sat: 6 g

1 3-ounce filet mignon
1/2 ounce Blue Castello triple cream cheese

Heat your oven to 500 degrees.
Heat an oven-tolerant grill on high, then sear the filet on one side, turning with tongs to make a cross hatch pattern on one side of the meat.
Turn the meat over and immediately place in the 500 degree oven. Cook 3 minutes for medium rare.
Serve the meat on a dish topped with a dab of cheese. Wait for it to melt before eating.

flank steak in adobo seasoning

1 1-1/2 pound flank steak, trimmed of any fat
3 to 4 cloves garlic, cut into slivers
adobo seasoning

Serves 6
per portion
Calories: 135
Protein: 14 g
Carbs: <1 g
Fat: 8 g
Sat: 3 g

Take flank steak and lightly score the surface on both sides in a criss-cross diamond pattern. Make slits in the meat and insert the slivers of garlic. Rub both sides of the meat with the adobo seasoning and place in a plastic bag in the refrigerator overnight.
Cook over a hot grill until the steak is rare inside and charred on the outside, about 7 to 9 minutes. Slice meat thinly across the grain.

I come from a family where
gravy is considered a beverage.
~Erma Bombeck~

grilled leg of lamb with rosemary and garlic

Serves 6
per portion
Calories: 169
Protein: 24 g
Carbs: 0 g
Fat: 8 g
Sat: 5 g

Have the butcher bone and butterfly the lamb, making cuts in the thickest parts and flattening the meat to uniform thickness. Make slits in the meat to insert slivers of garlic for a richer taste.

1/4 cup olive oil
1/3 cup dry red wine
1/4 cup red wine vinegar
1 tablespoon chopped fresh rosemary
3 garlic cloves, pressed
1 garlic clove, slice thinly
1-1/2 pounds deboned, butterflied leg of lamb

Mix first 5 ingredients in a large plastic bag.

Take the slices of garlic and push into the pockets in the meat.

Add the lamb to the marinade and refrigerate overnight, turning occasionally.

Prepare the barbecue on medium heat. Remove the lamb from the marinade and sprinkle with sea salt and pepper. Grill to desired doneness, about 20 minutes per side for medium rare, or roast in a 400 degree oven for 7 minutes for lamb medium rare.

Slice thinly and serve.

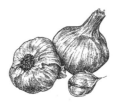

moorish spicy lamb kebabs

This is a heavily seasoned meat mixture that is best cooked over a charcoal grill. I was served this dish in Istanbul, while watching the sun gently lower into the sea behind the Blue Mosque.

Serves 8
per portion
Calories: 110
Protein: 12 g
Carbs: 1 g
Fat: 6 g
Sat: 2 g

2 garlic cloves, sliced
sea salt and black pepper
1 teaspoon coriander seeds
3/4 teaspoon paprika
3/4 teaspoon cumin seeds
1/2 teaspoon dried thyme
1/4 teaspoon crushed red pepper flakes
1 teaspoon curry powder
6 teaspoons olive oil
2 tablespoons lemon juice
1 tablespoon chopped fresh parsley
1 pound lean lamb, pork or beef,
    cut into 3/4 inch cubes

In a mortar, pound the garlic with a pinch of salt to make a paste.

Heat a skillet dry on high, then toast coriander seeds, cumin seeds, thyme, crushed red pepper and curry powder until hot and aromatic, about 30 seconds. Remove from the pan and put the mixture into a spice grinder until reduced to a fine powder.

In a bowl, combine the garlic, spices, olive oil, lemon juice, parsley, 3/4 teaspoon salt, pepper and the meat cubes. Toss well to coat completely and let marinate several hours, mixing occasionally.

Skewer the meat and grill over the coals, turning every 2-3 minutes, until well browned and still juicy, about 10 to 15 minutes. Baste occasionally with the marinade. Serve immediately.

pork chops with chipotle marinade

Serves 2
per portion
Calories: 130
Protein: 18 g
Carbs: 6 g
Fat: 3 g
Sat: 1 g

Today's pork is leaner than ever and lowers cholesterol better than poultry. If you like a fiery, hot dish, this seasoning will do the trick.

2 tablespoons canned chipotle peppers,
    including sauce
2 garlic cloves, crushed
1 3-inch strip of orange zest
1/4 cup fresh orange juice
1 tablespoon fresh lime juice
1/2 tablespoon red wine vinegar
3/4 teaspoon tomato paste
1/4 teaspoon dried Mexican oregano
1/4 teaspoon ground cumin
fresh pepper, sea salt to taste
2 3-ounce pork chops

In a small saucepan, combine the chipotles and their sauce with the garlic, orange zest, orange juice, lime juice, red wine vinegar, tomato paste, oregano, cumin and pepper. Simmer over high heat until reduced by one-third, about 3 minutes. Puree everything in a food processor until smooth. Let cool before using.

Place pork chops in a plastic bag and cover with the marinade. Refrigerate for 2 hours.

Grill on high heat for 5 minutes per side.

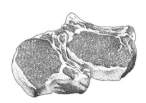

roast pork loin with garlic and rosemary

A classic French way to prepare a lean pork loin. Serve with fresh, steamed baby vegetables like zucchini or patty pan squash for a colorful presentation.

Serves 8
per portion
Calories: 218
Protein: 19 g
Carbs: 1 g
Fat: 15 g
Sat: 5 g

4 cloves garlic, pressed
4 teaspoons chopped fresh rosemary,
 or 2 teaspoons dried
1 1/2 teaspoons sea salt
1/2 teaspoon fresh Tellicherry black pepper
2 garlic cloves, sliced
2 1/2 pound boneless pork tenderloin roast,
 well trimmed

Preheat oven to 400 degrees. Line a 13x9x2 inch roasting pan with foil.

Mix first four ingredients together and rub all over the roast. Make small slits in the roast and stuff with the garlic slices.

Place pork fat side down in the roasting pan and roast for 30 minutes.

Turn roast fat side up and roast until thermometer inserted into the center of the pork loin registers 155 degrees, about 25 minutes longer.

Remove from the oven and let stand for 10 minutes before carving.

Pour pan juices over the pork slices and serve.

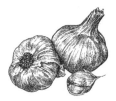

spicy beef with basil

*Serves 4
per portion
Calories: 108
Protein: 14 g
Carbs: 3 g
Fat: 4 g
Sat: 1 g*

There are numerous basils to choose from, but this dish cries out for its native Vietnamese basil, called holy basil. You can substitute Italian basil but you need to add mint leaves to try and approximate the unique flavor of holy basil. Look for it in any Far Eastern market.

1 teaspoon white peppercorns
2 garlic cloves, finely chopped
1 1/2 tablespoons coarsely chopped cilantro
1 tablespoon minced fresh ginger
2 Thai or serrano chilis, minced
1 1/2 teaspoons finely grated lime zest
1 teaspoon sea salt
1 teaspoon canola oil
8 ounces lean top round steak, cut into strips
2 tablespoons reduce sodium soy sauce
1 cup holy basil leaves, or 1/2 cup Italian basil
    and 1/2 cup mint leaves

Heat a small skillet dry on high heat, then toast the peppercorns until fragrant, about 1 minute. Transfer to a spice grinder and coarsely crush. In a bowl, add the garlic, cilantro, ginger, chilis, lime zest, peppercorns, sea salt and pound to a coarse paste.

Heat the skillet on high, then add the oil and reduce the heat to medium. Add the beef and stir-fry until cooked through, about 2 minutes. Stir in the soy sauce and transfer to serving bowls. Top with the basil.

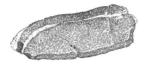

cuban grilled skirt steak

For this technique, it is easiest to partially freeze the skirt steak in order to slice it thin enough. If you substitute flank steak for skirt, you will need to slice it very thin or it will be tough.

Serves 2
per portion
Calories: 159
Protein: 15 g
Carbs: 7 g
Fat: 8 g
Sat: 4 g

1/2 small white onion, diced
1 serrano or jalapeno chili, diced
1/4 cup cilantro, chopped
1 garlic clove, minced
1 lime, juiced
2 teaspoons peanut oil
1/3 pound skirt steak

Combine onion, chili, cilantro, garlic and the juice of one lime in a non-reactive pan.

Partially freeze the skirt steak which has been trimmed of all fat. Using a very sharp knife, cut the steak in half horizontally. This may be done in sections, but the result will be a very thin cut of meat.

Combine the meat sections in the marinade for 15 minutes.

On a hot grill, quickly cook the meat until the edges are charred, turning only once. The meat will be medium rare inside.

Hunger finds no fault with the cook.
~ C.H.Spurgeon ~

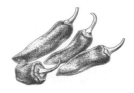

chapter nine

vegetables

aztec zucchini

This recipe comes from Emma Gonzalez, an Aztec raised in the mountains of Oaxaca. This is one of her most requested dishes. Do not substitute the type of mint or the oil as the flavor will not be the same.

2 teaspoons peanut oil
2 cans (14 1/2 ounces) Muir Glen tomatoes
1 clove garlic, chopped
1/4 white onion chopped
1 pound zucchini, sliced on the diagonal
1 tablespoon dried or 1/4 cup fresh spearmint,
    chopped
1/2 bunch cilantro, chopped

Serves 6
per portion
Calories: 95
Protein: 3 g
Carbs: 18 g
Fat: 2 g
Sat: <1 g

Heat an iron skillet dry on high heat, then add the peanut oil. Saute the tomatoes, garlic and onions until limp using a wooden spoon.

Add the zucchini, spearmint and cilantro and lower the heat. Cover and set on a low simmer for 15 minutes.

Cooking is like love.
It should be entered into
with abandon or not at all.
~Harriet Van Horne~

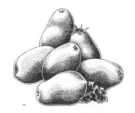

balsamic roasted squash and apples

Serves 4
per portion
Calories: 109
Protein: 2 g
Carbs: 26 g
Fat: 1 g
Sat: <1 g

This is another dish that comes alive with the unique pairing of balsamic and reduced apple cider glaze. I think you will find this dish is well worth the effort.

1/2 cup balsamic vinegar
1 cup fat free, reduced sodium chicken broth
few sprigs thyme
1 tablespoon apple cider glaze (see page 108)
2 (1- to 1-1/4 pound) acorn squash, halved
nonstick spray
2 green apples, peeled and cut into eighths
sea salt, pepper

Set the oven for 425 degrees.

Combine the vinegar, broth and thyme. Bring to a boil, then reduce the heat and simmer until the liquid is reduced to about 1/3 cup, about 15 minutes. Add the tablespoon of apple cider glaze and stir.

Remove the seeds from the squash and arrange the squash cut-side up in a single layer on a baking pan sprayed with nonstick cooking spray. Add the apples and brush with the balsamic glaze. Season with salt and pepper.

Roast until tender, about 35 minutes, brushing squash several times with the glaze.

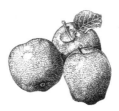

cauliflower leek puree

A great way to serve cauliflower is to puree it, adding another vegetable for flavor. Be sure to use only the white and pale green parts of the leeks and clean them carefully.

6 cups cauliflower, cut into pieces
1 cup chopped leeks
1 can fat free, reduced sodium chicken broth
sea salt, pepper

Serves 8
per portion
Calories: 33
Protein: 2 g
Carbs: 6 g
Fat: <1 g
Sat: 0 g

Place cauliflower, leeks and chicken broth in a microwave-safe bowl. Cover with plastic wrap and microwave on high for 14 minutes, or until vegetables are soft.
Transfer the vegetables to a food processor and blend until smooth. Add any cooking broth by tablespoons to achieve desired thickness and season with salt and pepper.

joel's asparagus bake

Joel is a very busy executive who finds time to cook only on the weekends. This is his easy, no holds barred approach for creating scrumptious, juicy asparagus every time. I like dipping it in menomaise for vegetables (p. 128).

Extra-virgin olive oil in a pump
1 pound asparagus, cleaned and trimmed
sea salt

Serves 2
per portion
Calories: 32
Protein: 6 g
Carbs: 3 g
Fat: <1 g
Sat: 0 g

Heat the oven to 400 degrees. Prepare the asparagus and place them flat in a lightly oiled glass dish. Do not bunch them up. Sprinkle with sea salt, spray with some additional oil and cover with foil.
Place in the oven on the middle rack and roast for 10 minutes. Remove the foil and roast an additional 10 minutes.

tuscany eggplant

Serves 6
per portion
Calories: 57
Protein: 2 g
Carbs: 10 g
Fat: 2 g
Sat: <1 g

I've never been a fan of eggplant, but this dish changed my mind. There's no need to salt the eggplant to extract any juice, so it's fast and easy to make.

2 teaspoons extra-virgin olive oil
1 onion, chopped
4 cloves garlic, minced
1 medium eggplant, peeled and chopped
2 green peppers, seeded and chopped
1 cup celery, chopped
5 Kalamata olives, chopped
1 cup mushrooms, chopped
1 can (8 ounces) tomato sauce
2 tablespoons red wine vinegar
1/4 teaspoon basil
sea salt, pepper

Heat skillet dry on high heat, then add the olive oil. Immediately lower the heat and saute the garlic and onion until tender. Add eggplant, green pepper and celery. Cover and cook for 15 minutes, stirring occasionally.

Add olives, mushrooms and tomato sauce, mixing thoroughly. Add vinegar and basil. Simmer uncovered until all ingredients are tender, about 15 minutes. Season with salt and pepper to taste. Serve warm.

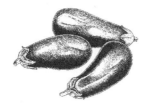

kabocha squash with tunisian flavors

Kabocha squash is a winter squash member that tastes sweet like pumpkin. It is used in Tunisia and Morocco. If you can't find it in your local grocery store, use butternut or pumpkin.

2 pounds kabocha squash
2 tablespoons water
1 head of garlic
1 teaspoon coriander
1/2 teaspoon cumin seeds
1/4 teaspoon caraway seeds
1 teaspoon sweet paprika
sea salt
pinch of cayenne
1 teaspoon fresh lemon juice

Serves 4
per portion
Calories: 50
Protein: 2 g
Carbs: 11 g
Fat: 1 g
Sat: 0 g

Preheat oven to 350 degrees. Cut the squash in half and scoop out the seeds. Set the halves, cut side down, on a lightly oiled baking sheet. Sprinkle the water on the pan. Pull the outer skin off the garlic, keeping the head intact. Wrap tightly in foil and place on the baking sheet. Bake until the squash is completely tender and the garlic feels soft, about 50 minutes. Let cool.

Scoop the squash flesh into the bowl of a food processor. Separate the garlic cloves and squeeze the pulp into the processor bowl.

In a small skillet, toast the coriander, cumin and caraway seeds over low heat until fragrant. Stir in the paprika. Transfer the spices to a mortar or spice grinder and let cool. Add 3/4 teaspoon salt and the cayenne and grind into a powder. Add half of the spice mix to the squash and process to a fine puree. Stir in more of the spice mix to taste. To serve, reheat the squash mixture in a pan sprayed with olive oil. Add the lemon juice and season with salt and pepper.

leeks nicoise

Serves 4
per portion
Calories: 109
Protein: 2 g
Carbs: 12 g
Fat: 7 g
Sat: 1 g

Here's another way to get onions into your diet. Leeks may contain dirt so be sure to split them at the bottom, make two deep cuts into the root and rinse well under water. Use a mandolin to finely slice the onions.

2 teaspoons extra-virgin olive oil
1 onion, thinly sliced
8 small leeks, cleaned
3 tomatoes, peeled and cut into eighths
1 garlic clove, crushed
1 tablespoon fresh basil, chopped
1 tablespoon fresh parsley, chopped
8 black olives, pitted and halved
sea salt, pepper
basil leaves to garnish

Heat a skillet dry on high then add the oil. Immediately reduce the heat and add the onions, cooking for 5 minutes or until soft. Add the leeks and cook, turning until just beginning to brown.

Add tomatoes. Stir in garlic, basil, parsley, olives, salt and pepper. Cover and cook over low heat 15 to 20 minutes or until leeks are tender, turning from time to time.

Remove leeks with a slotted spoon and transfer to a warm serving dish. Boil sauce for 2 minutes or until reduced and thickened. Pour over leeks and serve with basil leaves for garnish. May be presented hot or at room temperature.

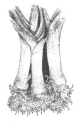

kabocha, fennel and orange casserole

I've always liked the combination of fennel and orange and this casserole makes a satisfying meal all in itself.

2 pounds kabocha squash, peeled, seeded
    and cut into 1-inch pieces
2 teaspoons extra-virgin olive oil
1 large white onion, chopped
4 celery stalks, chopped
1 large fennel bulb, trimmed and sliced fine
1/2 cup lentils
1 14-ounce can chopped tomatoes
1 cup fat free, reduced sodium chicken broth
sea salt, pepper
3 bay leaves
1 tablespoon chopped fresh sage
grated rind and chopped flesh of 2 oranges
1/3 cup walnuts

Serves 4
per portion
Calories: 230
Protein: 8 g
Carbs: 33 g
Fat: 9 g
Sat: 1 g

Heat a large pan on medium heat and add the oil. Cook the squash until it starts to soften, about 5 minutes. Stir in the onion, celery and fennel, reduce the heat and cook gently for 3 to 4 minutes, until soft.

Add the lentils, tomatoes and stock with all the seasonings and bring to boil. Reduce the heat and simmer gently for 30 minutes until the squash is tender.

Stir in the chopped orange, rind and nuts and cook for 2 more minutes. Remove the bay leaves and adjust the seasoning.

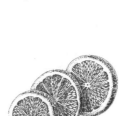

stir-fried bok choy

Serves 2
per portion
Calories: 29
Protein: 1 g
Carbs: 1 g
Fat: 2 g
Sat: <1 g

Known as Chinese cabbage, bok choy makes a wonderful vegetable to accompany pork dishes. Be sure and buy ones with dark green leaves as they contain lots of beta carotene. Here is an easy stir-fry version.

1 head bok choy
2 tablespoons water
1 1/2 teaspoons soy sauce, reduced salt
1 1/2 teaspoons oyster sauce
1 teaspoon peanut oil

Trim bok choy and cut crosswise into 1/4 inch slices.

In a bowl stir together water, soy and oyster sauces.

Heat dry a large heavy skillet or wok over high heat, then add oil and stir-fry boy choy for 2 minutes. Add the soy mixture and cook until crisp-tender, about 2 more minutes.

warm mixed greens

Serves 4
per portion
Calories: 87
Protein: 3 g
Carbs: 9 g
Fat: 6 g
Sat: 2 g

This is a delicious way to serve collard, kale, Swiss chard or mustard greens. For a slightly sweeter taste, add a tablespoon of reduced apple cider for a piquant flavor.

1 tablespoon unsalted butter
2 teaspoons extra-virgin olive oil
2 pounds braising greens trimmed and
    coarsely chopped
1 tablespoon reduced apple cider (p. 114)
2 tablespoons water
sea salt, pepper

In a large heavy saucepan, melt the butter in the olive oil. Add the greens, reduced apple cider and water and season with salt and pepper. Cover and cook over high heat until wilted and tender, about 2 to 3 minutes. Drain the greens and keep warm.

zucchini noodles with spicy tomato sauce

This is a fun dish. I used a Japanese mandolin that makes oodles of noodles out of any vegetable. For even more variety, alternate yellow and green squash. The splash of tomato sauce makes this dish "eye candy" for anyone lucky enough to have it placed before them.

Spicy Tomato Sauce
This will coat 1 pound of vegetable pasta
1 tablespoon extra-virgin olive oil
1/2 cup thinly sliced sweet onions
    (Vidalia, Walla Walla, Maui)
2 large garlic cloves, thinly sliced
2 14-1/2-ounce cans of Muir Glen peeled tomatoes
1/2 teaspoon crushed red pepper
sea salt
1 tablespoon minced spearmint

Heat a large skillet dry on high heat then add oil. Immediately lower the heat and add the onion and cook, stirring, until softened and just brown, about 5 minutes. Stir in the garlic and cook for 1 minute. Add the tomatoes with their juice and the crushed red pepper. Season with salt and cook, stirring, until thickened, about 20 minutes. Stir in the mint.

Makes 2 1/2 cups
per 1/2 cup
Calories: 43
Protein: 1 g
Carbs: 6 g
Fat: 2 g
Sat: <1 g

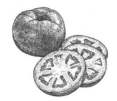

zucchini noodles

Serves 4
per portion
Calories: 50
Protein: 1 g
Carbs: 4 g
Fat: 4 g
Sat: <1 g

If you want to save time or don't have a Japanese mandolin, use spaghetti squash and bake according to directions. To save even more time and calories, blanch the "noodles" in boiling water for 2 minutes and drain.

1 tablespoon extra-virgin olive oil
1 1/2 teaspoons thyme leaves
1 teaspoon minced garlic
1 1/2 pounds zucchini, yellow squash,
    finely shredded into noodles
sea salt, pepper

In a large skillet, warm the olive oil and add half the thyme and all the garlic and cook over moderate heat for 1 minute. Add the zucchini and cook, stirring occasionally, until it just begins to lose its crunch, about 3 minutes. Season with salt and pepper.
Top with the spicy tomato sauce.

I never see any home cooking.
All I get is fancy stuff.
~Duke of Edinburgh~

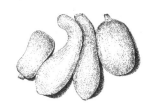

roasted sweet red peppers

I often make jars of roasted peppers to have on hand when I want a really great snack. They go especially well with goat cheese and basil.

4 to 6 medium red peppers
2 garlic cloves, minced
2 tablespoons red wine vinegar
2 teaspoons extra-virgin olive oil
sea salt
2 tablespoons chopped fresh basil

Roast the peppers over a flame until charred and blistered. Set in a paper bag and let cool. Remove the skins. Split the peppers in half and remove the seeds and inner membranes. Cut the peppers into wide strips.

Place in a bowl and toss with the garlic, vinegar, olive oil and salt to taste. Cover and refrigerate until ready to serve. Do not add the basil until ready to serve.

Serves 4-6
per portion
Calories: 40
Protein: 1 g
Carbs: 4 g
Fat: 2 g
Sat: 0 g

Chili is a lot like sex:
when it's good it's great,
and even when it's bad, it's not bad.
~ Bill Boldenweck ~

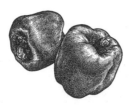

chapter ten

cereals, grains and beans

connemara irish oatmeal

bahian black bean chili

black beans with garlic, cilantro and cumin

garbanzos with garlic and kale

lima beans with chives

rosemary and lemon pinto beans

pumpkin and navy bean cassoulet

red lentil and tofu curry

connemara irish oatmeal

My daughter and I took a trip to Ireland where we explored the countryside and frightened quite a few natives with my driving. We were served this wonderful oatmeal which I have adapted to include a portion of soy. It's better than any lucky charm!

1/3 cup Irish cut oats
1/2 cup soy milk
1 tablespoon whey protein powder
2 packets Nutrasweet™

Place milk and Irish oats in a saucepan and bring to a boil. Reduce the heat and simmer for twenty minutes until soft but still liquid. It will thicken as it stands.
Blend in the sweetener.

Serves 1
per portion
Calories: 304
Protein: 20 g
Carbs: 43 g
Fat: 7 g
Sat: 2 g

Only dull people are brilliant at breakfast.
~ Oscar Wilde ~

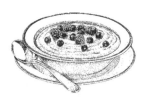

bahian black bean chili

Serves 8
per portion
Calories: 221
Protein: 9 g
Carbs: 38 g
Fat: 3 g
Sat: <1 g

While presenting at a conference in Rio de Janeiro, I was treated to a Brazilian dinner in the home of a friend. His wife prepared this chili which was even better the next morning for breakfast. For an extra kick, try adding sweet Spanish smoked paprika. Your family will love the samba beat it puts in your step.

4 teaspoons extra-virgin olive oil
1 clove garlic, minced
2 medium yellow onions, diced
1 medium poblano chili, diced
2 tablespoons cumin seed
2 tablespoons oregano
1 teaspoon cayenne pepper
1 1/2 teaspoons paprika
1 teaspoon sea salt
1/2 cup jalapeno chili, chopped with seeds
2 15-ounce cans black beans
24 ounces Muir Glen organic tomatoes, crushed
5 teaspoons soy powder
8 sprigs cilantro plus 2 tablespoons chopped
1/2 cup green onions, finely chopped
8 tablespoons white vinegar
2 medium oranges

Heat an iron skillet dry on high heat, then add the olive oil and saute the garlic, onions and poblano chili on medium heat until soft.

Add the cumin, oregano, cayenne pepper, paprika and sea salt to the mixture along with the tomatoes and chili and saute for 10 minutes on low heat.

Add the beans, soy and chopped cilantro and stir.

To serve, place the hot chili in a heated bowl, and sprinkle with some green onion. Float a tablespoon of vinegar on the top.

Cut oranges into quarters and serve alongside the chili.

black beans with garlic, cilantro and cumin

This dish is typical of the Latin style of preparing black beans. It's quick, easy and the fragrance will make you yearn for a cabana on the beach.

15 ounces black beans, canned
2 garlic cloves
1 teaspoon ground cumin
1 teaspoon extra-virgin olive oil
1/3 cup tomato juice
3/4 teaspoon sea salt
2 tablespoons chopped cilantro

Rinse the black beans and drain. Chop the garlic. In a nonstick skillet cook garlic and cumin in oil over moderate heat, stirring, until fragrant. Add black beans, juice, salt and cook, stirring until beans are heated through. Stir in cilantro and serve.

Serves 4
per portion
Calories: 155
Protein: 8 g
Carbs: 24 g
Fat: 2 g
Sat: <1 g

Garlic is the catsup of intellectuals.
~Anonymous~

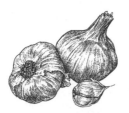

garbanzos with garlic and kale

Serves 6
per portion
Calories: 122
Protein: 6 g
Carbs: 22 g
Fat: 2 g
Sat: <1 g

During a trip to Hong Kong, I tasted this dish at a little sidewalk shop that was filled with locals. I think you will agree it has a unique, filling taste.

2 bunches kale or collard greens
1 teaspoon extra-virgin olive oil
4 cloves garlic
1 tablespoon minced gingerrroot
1 red chili pepper, finely chopped
2 tomatoes, coarsely chopped
1 15-ounce can garbanzo beans, including liquid
1 teaspoon reduced sodium soy sauce
1 teaspoon hoisin sauce

Wash the kale, remove the stems and chop the leaves.

Heat the oil in a large skillet and saute the garlic, gingerroot and pepper for 2 minutes.

Stir in the tomatoes and garbanzo beans with their liquid. Bring to a simmer and cook for 5 minutes.

Add the soy sauce, hoisin sauce and stir to mix. Spread the kale evenly over the top, then cover the pan and cook over medium heat, stirring occasionally, until the kale is tender, about 5 to 7 minutes. Do not overcook.

lima beans with chives

2 cups frozen lima beans
Water to cover beans
1 small onion, studded with 3 whole cloves
5 whole Tellicherry black peppercorns
1 thyme sprig
1 bay leaf
1/4 cup water
1 tablespoon extra-virgin olive oil
sea salt
2 tablespoons fresh minced chives

Serves 8
per portion
Calories: 60
Protein: 2 g
Carbs: 8 g
Fat: 2 g
Sat: <1 g

   Place the beans in a microwave safe container and add water to cover the beans, onion, peppercorns, thyme and bay leaf. Microwave on high for 5 minutes. Drain the beans, discarding the spices. Chop the onion into pieces and add to the beans.
   In a large skillet, combine the beans with 1/4 cup water and cook over moderately high heat, stirring, for 2 minutes. Add the olive oil, season with salt and pepper, sprinkle with the chives and serve.

rosemary and lemon pinto beans

1 15-ounce can pinto beans, rinsed and drained
1/3 cup thinly sliced red onion
1 teaspoon extra-virgin olive oil
1 tablespoon red wine vinegar
1 teaspoon minced fresh rosemary
1 garlic clove, minced
Dash hot pepper sauce

Serves 4
per portion
Calories: 96
Protein: 5 g
Carbs: 16 g
Fat: 1 g
Sat: <1 g

   Combine the ingredients in a bowl and toss to blend. Season to taste with salt and pepper.

pumpkin and navy bean cassoulet

Serves 6
per portion
Calories: 157
Protein: 8 g
Carbs: 28 g
Fat: 3 g
Sat: <1 g

Pumpkin is available all year round and is an excellent source for fiber and beta carotene. If you can't find fresh pumpkin, use a butternut squash.

1 can navy beans
2 teaspoons extra-virgin olive oil
2 medium white onions, sliced
2 pounds pumpkin or butternut squash
2 garlic cloves, sliced
3 zucchini, cut into 1-inch pieces
sea salt, pepper
1 14-ounce can Muir Glen tomatoes, chopped
4 large sprigs thyme
3 bay leaves

Drain the beans and rinse.
Preheat the oven to 325 degrees.
Heat a pan dry on high heat, then add the olive oil and immediately reduce the heat. Cook the onions until softened, then stir in the pumpkin, garlic and zucchini. Adjust the seasoning and pour the mixture into an ovenproof casserole dish. Pour the tomatoes over top and place the thyme and bay leaves into the mixture. Top with the beans and add enough water to come just below the level of the beans. Cover and cook for 45 minutes.

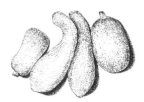

red lentil and tofu curry

Red lentils are actually orange, but they create a creamy base when cooked. Lentils supply a hefty dose of fiber, protein, complex carbohydrate and impressive complements of iron, thiamin, niacin, phosphorus and potassium.

Serves 4
per portion
Calories: 136
Protein: 10 g
Carbs: 19 g
Fat: 3 g
Sat: <1 g

1 small yellow onion
1 garlic clove
1/2 inch piece of fresh gingerroot
1/2 cup red lentils, uncooked
1 teaspoon canola oil
3 1/2 cups water
1/2 cup firm tofu
1/2 teaspoon cumin seeds
1/2 teaspoon garam masala or curry powder
    (see Resources)
1/2 teaspoon sea salt
Pinch of cayenne
cilantro to garnish

Thinly slice onion and mince garlic. Peel gingerroot and mince. In a sieve, rinse lentils, removing any stones, and drain.

In a 2 quart heavy saucepan cook onion and garlic in 1 teaspoon oil over moderate heat, stirring until golden. Add gingerroot and cook, stirring, 1 minute. Add lentils and water and gently bring to a boil, uncovered, until lentils fall apart, about 20 minutes.

While lentils are boiling, rinse and drain tofu and cut into small squares.

In a heavy skillet, spray with oil and cook cumin seeds, stirring until a shade darker, about 1 minute. Add garam masala, salt, and cayenne and cook, stirring, until fragrant, 15 to 30 seconds. Stir hot spice oil into the lentils and gently stir in the tofu cubes. Let curry stand, covered, 5 minutes to allow flavors to develop. Sprinkle with cilantro and serve.

chapter eleven

fruits and desserts

white sangria splash

winter fruit salad

yellow tomato, watermelon
and arugula salad

fruit with string cheese

spicy fruit salad

strawberries with cassis, balsamic vinegar
and mint

apple in dutch chocolate

kir royale mold

roasted peaches with cardamom

white sangria splash

This recipe comes from the JELL-O people and makes a sophisticated dessert that's low in calories yet packed with fruit. If you use mineral water you can get your calcium too!

1 cup dry white wine
1 package (8 serving size) JELL-O brand
      lemon flavor sugar free low calorie gelatin dessert
3 cups cold club soda or mineral water
1 tablespoon lime juice
1 tablespoon orange juice
1 cup green and/or red grapes
1 cup sliced strawberries
1 cup yogurt
2 tablespoons whipping cream

Serves 8
per portion
Calories: 82
Protein: 3 g
Carbs: 8 g
Fat: 2 g
Sat: 1 g

Bring the wine to boil in a small saucepan. Stir boiling wine into gelatin in a medium bowl at least 2 minutes until completely dissolved. Stir in the club soda, lime juice and orange juice. Reserve one cup of the gelatin at room temperature.

Place the bowl of gelatin in a larger bowl of ice water. Let stand about 10 minutes or until thickened, stirring occasionally. If the spoon drawn through the mixture leaves definite impressions, it is ready for the next step.

Add the grapes and strawberries. Pour into three 2 cup molds or one 6 cup mold. Refrigerate about 2 hours or until set but not firm (should stick to your finger).

Stir the yogurt and whipping cream into the reserved gelatin with a wire whisk until smooth. Pour over the gelatin mold.

Refrigerate 4 hours or until firm. Unmold. Garnish as desired.

winter fruit salad

Serves 4
per portion
Calories: 77
Protein: 1 g
Carbs: 14 g
Fat: 3 g
Sat: <1 g

I have a lovely kumquat tree in my backyard that yields fruit nearly year round, but especially in the winter. This salad is colorful and has a great flavor.

6 kumquats, halved, seeded and coarsely chopped
2 tablespoons coarsely chopped cilantro
2 teaspoons extra-virgin olive oil
2-1/2 tablespoons fresh squeezed lemon juice
2-1/2 tablespoons coarsely chopped cilantro
1/2 teaspoon sea salt
1 large Bosc pear, peeled,
    cored and cut into 1/2-inch dice
1 medium cucumber, peeled,
    seeded and cut into 1/2-inch dice
1 cup coarsely chopped stemmed watercress

In a small bowl, combine the kumquats and cilantro with the olive oil, lemon juice and salt and let steep for 5 minutes.

In a large bowl, toss together the pear and cucumber and add the dressing and toss well. Add the watercress and toss again.

I'm like certain kinds of fruit:
bitter outside and sweet inside.
~Sharon Stone~

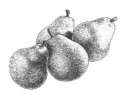

yellow tomato, watermelon and arugula salad

Finally, a tomato you can pop into your mouth without fear of squishing seeds out the side. Look for these teardrop tomatoes in both red and yellow in your local farmer's market or grocery store. It's a great way to put more lycopene, a chemical that fights cancer, in your diet.

Serves 4
per portion
Calories: 48
Protein: 1 g
Carbs: 6 g
Fat: 3 g
Sat: <1 g

3/4 cup watermelon, cubed
2 tablespoon balsamic vinegar
2 teaspoons extra-virgin olive oil
2 ounces arugula leaves, large stems removed
3/4 pound yellow teardrop tomatoes, sliced in half

In a medium bowl, toss the watermelon cubes with one tablespoon of the vinegar and season with salt and pepper. Let stand for 5 minutes, then drain.

In a small bowl, whisk the remaining tablespoon of vinegar with the olive oil and toss with the arugula. Mix together the tomatoes, watermelon and salad and serve.

fruit with string cheese

I keep small individual packages of string cheese to eat with any fruit.

Serves 1
per portion
Calories: 178
Protein: 8 g
Carbs: 25 g
Fat: 7 g
Sat: 0 g

1 package string cheese
1 pear

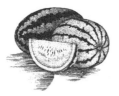

spicy fruit salad

Serves 8
per portion
Calories: 106
Protein: 2 g
Carbs: 26 g
Fat: 1 g
Sat: 0 g

1 16-ounce can sliced peaches
2 3-inch-long cinnamon sticks
   (use Mexican cinnamon if available)
3/4 teaspoon ground allspice
2 large navel oranges
2 large pink grapefruits
1 small pineapple
2 pints strawberries
3 kiwifruits
2 tablespoons chopped crystallized ginger

Drain syrup from peaches into small saucepan. Place peaches in large bowl.

Over medium-high heat, heat syrup, cinnamon, and ground allspice to boiling.

Reduce heat to low; cover and simmer 10 minutes. Set syrup mixture aside to cool while preparing fruit.

Grate peel from 1 orange; set aside. Cut peel from oranges and grapefruits.

To catch juice, hold fruit over bowl with peaches and cut sections from oranges and grapefruits between membranes; drop sections into bowl.

Cut peel and core from pineapple; cut fruit into 1 1/2-inch chunks. Add pineapple to fruit in bowl.

Pour syrup mixture over fruit in bowl. Add grated orange peel; toss.

Cover and refrigerate until ready to serve.

Just before serving, hull strawberries; cut strawberries in half if large. Cut peel from kiwifruits. Slice each kiwifruit lengthwise into 6 wedges. Toss strawberries and kiwifruits with fruit mixture. Place fruit salad in serving bowl. Sprinkle with crystallized ginger.

strawberries with cassis, balsamic vinegar and mint

This is an ingenious Italian dessert that presents a rich sweet and sour taste. I first enjoyed this at the La Varenne Cooking School in Paris.

1 pound strawberries
2 tablespoons creme de cassis
1 tablespoon balsamic vinegar
6 large mint leaves, cut into slices
black pepper

Serves 4
per portion
Calories: 92
Protein: 1 g
Carbs: 16 g
Fat: 1 g
Sat: 0 g

Cut the berries in half.

Toss with the creme de cassis and refrigerate, covered for one hour or more.

Just before serving, toss with the balsamic vinegar and mint. Crack fresh pepper over top.

apple in dutch chocolate

Gillian Anderson gave this secret away. Any fruit will do, but Fuji or Gala apples seem the tastiest when dipped in this chocolate powder.

1 Fuji or Gala apple
1 package Swiss Miss™ Diet Hot Cocoa Mix

Serves 1
per portion
Calories: 101
Protein: 2 g
Carbs: 25 g
Fat: <1 g
Sat: 0 g

Cut apple into wedges. Do not peel.

Rip package of hot cocoa mix open. Hold in your non-dominant hand.

Carefully dip the apple wedges into the mix and enjoy!

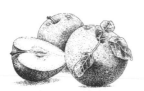

kir royale mold

Serves 8
per portion
Calories: 38
Protein: 2 g
Carbs: 4 g
Fat: 2 g
Sat: 1 g

2 cups boiling water
1 package (8 serving size) JELL-O brand
   Sparkling White Grape sugar free low
   calorie gelatin dessert
1 1/2 cups club soda or mineral water
2 tablespoons creme de cassis liqueur
1 tablespoon whipping cream
2 cups raspberries

Stir the boiling water into the gelatin in a large bowl at least 2 minutes until completely dissolved. Refrigerate 15 minutes.

Gently stir in the cold club soda, liqueur and whipping cream. Refrigerate for 30 minutes or until slightly thickened (the consistency of unbeaten egg whites). Gently stir for 15 seconds and add the raspberries.

Pour into a 6 cup mold and refrigerate for 4 hours or until firm. Unmold and garnish as desired.

When you get to fifty-two,
food becomes more important than sex.
~ Prue Leith ~

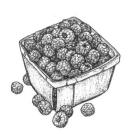

roasted peaches with cardamom

I never knew that roasting peaches could taste so good. Just inhale the fragrance as you serve them and you'll think you're lost in an orchard in Georgia.

Serves 6
per portion
Calories: 78
Protein: 1 g
Carbs: 11 g
Fat: 4 g
Sat: 1 g

6 ripe, firm peaches
1 tablespoon lemon juice
1 tablespoon unsalted butter
1 cinnamon stick, broken into 3 pieces
pinch of ground cloves
1 tablespoon ground cardamom
1 tablespoon grated lemon zest
3 tablespoons almond slices
1 small bunch mint leaves

Preheat oven to 400 degrees.

Dip the peaches in a pot of boiling water for 30 seconds, then place in ice water. Remove from the water and peel the skin. Quarter the peaches, removing the pits. Gently rub with lemon juice to prevent discoloration.

Melt the butter in large saucepan and add the cinnamon, cloves, cardamom and lemon zest. Cook over low heat for about 15 minutes, stirring occasionally. Add the peaches to the spicy butter, toss gently and transfer to a roasting pan. Bake for 15 minutes.

Arrange on a platter, sprinkle almonds and mint on top of the fruit.

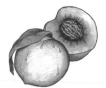

chapter twelve
seasonings and rubs

These are recipes for seasonings that can make any simple dish a gourmet delight. I keep them on hand for grilling and they really bring out the flavor of poultry when placed under the skin.

adobo seasoning

2 tablespoons Pasilla chili powder
2 tablespoons paprika
5 teaspoons Mexican oregano
1 tablespoon ground cumin
1 tablespoon ground mustard
2 tablespoons sea salt
3/4 teaspoon cayenne pepper

Combine seasoning in a bowl. Store in a covered container.

arkansas spice rub

2 tablespoons ground cumin
1 tablespoon chili powder
1 tablespoon dry mustard
1 tablespoon coarse sea salt
1 1/2 teaspoons cayenne pepper
1 1/2 teaspoons ground cardamom
1 1/2 teaspoons ground cinnamon

Combine all in a bowl and use to rub on meats.

The larger the pepper mill,
the lousier the food.
~ Mike Kalina ~

california bbq seasoning

I have used this seasoning combination on ribs and chicken with no complaints from any of my guests. I often place it under the skin of a turkey or chicken for extra flavor.

1 cup of kosher salt
1/2 cup garlic powder
3 tablespoons cayenne
1 tablespoon white pepper
1 tables black pepper
1 teaspoon onion powder

danish rub

This spice combination is especially good on salmon if you are preparing graavlax or lox.

3 tablespoons whole coriander seeds
3 tablespoons dill seeds
3 tablespoons yellow mustard seeds
6 tablespoons whole fennel seeds
3 tablespoons sea salt
1 1/2 teaspoons Tellicherry black peppercorns

Combine all the seeds in a skillet over medium heat, shaking the pan until aromatic, about 4 minutes.

Using a spice grinder, coarsely grind seeds. Add salt and peppercorns and grind again. Keeps at room temperature in an airtight container for up to 6 months.

Salt is born of the purest of parents:
the sun and the sea.
~Pythagoras~

italian seasoning

I first enjoyed this seasoning at Tra Vigne restaurant in Napa Valley. It was served on their grilled roast chicken. You will never eat plain chicken again after tasting this.

1 cup sea salt or kosher salt
3 tablespoons Pasilla chile powder (see Resources)
2 tablespoons Ancho chile powder (see Resources)
1 tablespoon fennel
1 tablespoon cumin
1 teaspoon coriander

Grind in spice mill and store in a covered container.

moroccan seasoning

1 tablespoon paprika
1 teaspoon turmeric
1/2 teaspoon cumin
1/2 teaspoon cinnamon
1/2 teaspoon ginger

Blend and use with any liquid to baste fish or poultry.

*If the doctors of today will not become
the nutritionists of tomorrow,
the nutritionists of today will become
the doctors of tomorrow.*
~ Thomas Edison ~

tunisian seasoning

1 teaspoon sea salt
1/4 teaspoon cumin seeds
1/4 teaspoon coriander seeds
1/4 teaspoon fennel seeds
1/4 teaspoon Aleppo pepper (see Resources)
1/8 teaspoon nigella (see Resources)

Place in a spice grinder and blend. Store in an airtight container.

ras el hanout

This is the "top of the shop" spice mixture from Morocco. In its classic form it has 27 spices, but here is a much simpler version. You can also obtain various mixtures by direct mail (see Resources).

1 teaspoon cumin seeds
1 teaspoon ginger
1 1/2 teaspoons coriander seeds
1 1/2 teaspoons black peppercorns
     (preferably Tellicherry)
1/4 teaspoon cayenne pepper
4 whole cloves
6 allspice berries
1 1/2 teaspoons ground cinnamon
     (preferably Mexican)

Grind in a spice mill and store in an airtight jar.

reduced apple cider

This is a great base to have on hand whenever a recipe calls for honey. By reducing apple cider, you have a concentrate that works equally well as a glaze for meat, in sauces and in salad dressings. Do not use sparkling cider.

1 gallon apple cider

In a large saucepan, boil the cider over high heat until reduced to 1 quart, about 1 1/2 hours. Reduce the heat to moderate and simmer until further reduced to the consistency of maple syrup, about 45 minutes. Let the cider cool completely, then store in a tightly sealed jar in the refrigerator. It will keep indefinitely.

Makes 2 cups
per tablespoon
Calories: 53
Protein: <1 g
Carbs: 13 g
Fat: <1 g
Sat: 0 g

An apple is an excellent thing—
until you have tried a peach!
~ George du Maurier ~

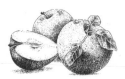

chapter thirteen

sauces, salsas and dressings

ancho-sun dried tomato pesto

This is great with pork or chicken and is easy to make. Sun dried tomatoes have a wonderful flavor and keep forever in a cool, dark place, so keep some on hand in your pantry.

4 large, dried ancho chilis, stemmed, seeded,
    torn into pieces (see Resources)
4 sun-dried tomatoes (not in oil), chopped
2/3 cup chopped roasted red peppers from a jar
2 tablespoons apple cider vinegar
1 tablespoon extra-virgin olive oil
1 tablespoon sesame seeds

Serves 12
per portion
Calories: 48
Protein: 2 g
Carbs: 7 g
Fat: 2 g
Sat: <1 g

Place chilis and tomatoes in a medium metal bowl and add enough boiling water to cover; let soften 20 minutes. Drain chilis and tomatoes, reserving 3/4 cup soaking liquid. Transfer chilis, tomatoes and reserved liquid to blender. Add remaining ingredients; blend until smooth. Season with salt and pepper.

Can be made 2 days ahead. Cover and chill.

Pesto is the quiche of the '80s.
~Nora Ephron~

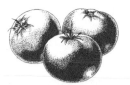

tomato and caper sauce

Serves 4
per portion
Calories: 54
Protein: 2 g
Carbs: 7 g
Fat: 3 g
Sat: <1 g

This is excellent served over fish or grilled chicken. Capers give a wonderful, piquant flavor to tomatoes so keep a jar handy in the refrigerator.

2 teaspoons extra-virgin olive oil
1 tablespoon minced, fresh garlic
2 tablespoons capers
2 cups cored and chopped fresh
    or drained canned tomatoes
Basil leaves, minced or chiffonade style
sea salt, black pepper

Heat olive oil in a medium-to-large skillet over medium heat. Add the garlic and cook until lightly colored, being careful not to burn the garlic.

Add the capers and cook for 15 seconds, then add the tomatoes and cook until thick, about 10 minutes. Season with salt and pepper.

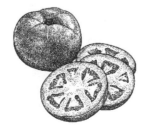

citrus salsa

In New Zealand, my friends Helen and Richard took me to a small, local restaurant in the Wairarapa that served this salsa over fish. I even enjoy it as a salad.

1 English cucumber, seeded and diced
2 red bell peppers, seeded and diced
1 small red onion, diced
1 jalapeno chili, diced
1 tablespoon capers
2 limes, zested
2 navel oranges, zested
1 tablespoon chopped fresh mint leaves
2 tablespoons extra-virgin olive oil
sea salt

   Combine the diced cucumber, pepper, onion and jalapeno chili in a non-reactive bowl. Drain the capers. Finely grate the zest from the limes and oranges and cut the citrus sections free from the membranes and cut into 1/2-inch pieces. Combine all the ingredients, toss and season with salt.

Serves 12
per portion
Calories: 47
Protein: 1 g
Carbs: 7 g
Fat: 2 g
Sat: <1 g

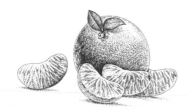

chili verde sauce

Serves 12
per portion
1/3 cup
Calories: 23
Protein: 0 g
Carbs: 3 g
Fat: 1 g
Sat: 0 g

Another of Emma's great sauces from Oaxaca. Watch for tomatillos in season as they are sweeter than canned. The sticky paper wrapping around them comes off easily if you rinse them under water first. If you serve this sauce over chicken, turkey or pork, just stand back and accept the applause.

1 pound green tomatillos in the husk
1 serrano chili with seeds
2 cloves of garlic
1 bunch of cilantro
1/4 white onion, chopped
1 teaspoon of cumin whole seeds
2 teaspoons peanut oil
sea salt

Steam tomatillos and chilis for twenty minutes. Cool.

Place the tomatillos, chilis, garlic, cilantro, onion and cumin in the blender on lowest setting. Once the initial chopping is done, blend on high.

Heat an iron skillet dry on high heat, then add the peanut oil and pour the mixture into the skillet. Immediately reduce the heat and simmer, uncovered until the desired consistency.

Season with sea salt.

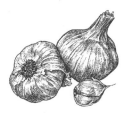

tarragon chive sauce

1/2 cup mayonnaise, reduced fat
1/3 cup fresh tarragon leaves
1-1/3 cup yogurt
3 tablespoons finely chopped chives
1 teaspoon lime juice
sea salt, pepper

Makes 2 cups
per tablespoon
Calories: 37
Protein: 1 g
Carbs: 1 g
Fat: 3 g
Sat: 1 g

   In a food processor pulse together mayonnaise, tarragon and 1/3 cup of the yogurt until smooth. Transfer mixture to a bowl and stir in remaining cup yogurt, chives, lime juice and salt and pepper to taste. Garnish with chives.

yogurt, chive and dijon mustard dressing

1/3 cup whole milk yogurt
3 tablespoons Dijon mustard
2 tablespoons reduced-fat mayonnaise
1 bunch fresh chopped chives

Serves 4
per portion
Calories: 53
Protein: 2 g
Carbs: 2 g
Fat: 4 g
Sat: 1 g

   In a small bowl whisk together all the dressing ingredients. Chill, covered for 1 day.

So far I've kept my diet secret,
but now I might as well tell everyone what it is.
Lots of grapefruit throughout the day
and plenty of virile young men at night.
~ Angie Dickinson ~

tomatillo celery salsa

Makes 3 cups
per 3/4 cup
Calories: 36
Protein: <1 g
Carbs: 7 g
Fat: 0 g
Sat: 0 g

1 pound fresh tomatillos
4 celery ribs
1 cup packed fresh cilantro sprigs
6 radishes
1 tablespoon fresh lemon juice

Remove husks and wash tomatillos under warm water to remove stickiness. Pat dry and cut about three fourths into 1/4-inch dice.

In a blender puree remaining tomatillos until smooth.

Cut celery into 1/4-inch dice and finely chop cilantro. Slice radishes and cut into julienne strips.

In a bowl toss together all ingredients and season with salt.

walnut and sage sauce

Makes 1 cup
per tablespoon
Calories: 48
Protein: 1 g
Carbs: 1 g
Fat: 5 g
Sat: <1 g

In the Basque region, walnuts are a local product, and cooks on the Spanish side of the border often make nut sauces like this one. Use it to dress pork or lamb dishes.

1/3 cup walnuts
1/3 cup whole almonds
1 small clove garlic
1/2 teaspoon coriander seeds
2 tablespoons extra-virgin olive oil

In a food processor, combine the walnuts, almonds, garlic and coriander seeds and add 1/4 cup olive oil. Pulse just until the mixture resembles a coarse pesto.

watermelon, cantaloupe and red pepper salsa

3/4 pound watermelon, diced
1/2 pound cantaloupe, diced
1/2 red bell pepper
1/2 small sweet onion (Vidalia, Maui, Walla Walla)
1/3 cup packed fresh cilantro sprigs
1/2 fresh jalapeno chili
2 tablespoons chopped fresh spearmint leaves
1 tablespoon fresh lime juice
sea salt

Makes 4 cups
per cup
Calories: 59
Protein: 1 g
Carbs: 13 g
Fat: <1 g
Sat: 0 g

Remove rinds and seeds from the melons and cut fruit into 1/4-inch dice. Devein and deseed bell pepper and cut into 1/4-inch dice.

Finely chop onion, cilantro and jalapeno chili, including the seeds.

In a bowl, combine all the ingredients and season with sea salt.

white wine sauce with grapes and tarragon

2 teaspoons extra-virgin olive oil
2 medium shallots, minced
1 tablespoon chopped fresh tarragon leaves
1/2 cup dry white wine
1 cup seedless grapes, halved lengthwise
1/2 cup fat free, reduced sodium chicken broth
sea salt, pepper

Serves 4
per portion
Calories: 63
Protein: 1 g
Carbs: 5 g
Fat: 2 g
Sat: <1 g

Heat pan over medium heat and add olive oil. Saute shallots until softened, about 1 minute. Add tarragon, wine and grapes; increase heat to medium-high and bring to a boil. Cook until reduced and syrupy, 4 to 5 minutes.

Add chicken broth, stirring occasionally until thickened and reduced to 3/4 cup, about 4 minutes. Adjust seasoning.

navy bean, garlic and tomato salsa

Makes 4 cups
per 1/3 cup
Calories: 54
Protein: 3 g
Carbs: 12 g
Fat: <1 g
Sat: 0 g

1 head garlic
1 16-ounce can navy beans
3 medium vine-ripened tomatoes
   (about 1-1/4 pounds)
1 small sweet onion (Vidalia, Walla Walla, Maui)
1/2 cup packed fresh basil leaves
2 tablespoons fresh lemon juice
sea salt

Preheat oven to 400 degrees.

Cut off the top of a head of garlic, wrap in foil and bake for 30 minutes. Unwrap garlic and cool. Peel skins from each clove and in a bowl mash the garlic pulp until smooth.

Rinse and drain enough beans to measure 1 cup and add to the garlic.

Cut 2 tomatoes into 1/4-inch dice and add to the beans. Quarter remaining tomato and in a blender puree until smooth. Add puree to the bean mixture.

Finely chop onion and basil and add to the bean mixture with lemon juice, tossing to combine. Season salsa with sea salt and pepper.

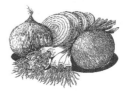

blood orange citrus dressing

There's plenty of zing in this dressing, which can grace a fruit salad just as easily as any greens. I especially like it over watermelon, oranges, watercress and mint. Throw in some red onion slices and you have a real treat!

2 tablespoons fresh lemon juice
1 tablespoon blood orange juice
2 teaspoons whole-grain Dijon mustard
1 teaspoon grated blood orange peel
3 teaspoons extra-virgin olive oil

Whisk first 5 ingredients in a small bowl to blend. Gradually add oil and whisk until combined. Season with salt and pepper to taste.

Serves 6
per portion
Calories: 24
Protein: <1 g
Carbs: <1 g
Fat: 2 g
Sat: <1 g

dijon balsamic vinaigrette

Cordon Bleu teaches a trick to keep an emulsion, like this recipe, intact—beat it with a little birch whisk. The oils from the branches let you make this dressing long in advance without fear of it separating. Can't find enough birch branches? Just blend with a whisk and serve immediately.

2 teaspoons Dijon mustard
1 tablespoon balsamic vinegar
2 tablespoons extra-virgin olive oil
1 teaspoon finely chopped fresh tarragon leaves
sea salt, pepper

In a small bowl whisk together mustard and vinegar. Add the oil in a slow stream, whisking until emulsified. Whisk in tarragon and salt and pepper to taste.

Serves 4
per portion
Calories: 62
Protein: <1 g
Carbs: <1 g
Fat: 7 g
Sat: 1 g

fennel-tarragon vinaigrette

Serves 8
per portion
Calories: 51
Protein: <1 g
Carbs: <1 g
Fat: 6 g
Sat: 1 g

2 tablespoons white wine vinegar
4 teaspoons chopped fresh tarragon
2 teaspoons Dijon mustard
1 teaspoon fennel seeds, crushed
3-1/3 tablespoons extra-virgin olive oil

Whisk first 4 ingredients in a medium bowl to blend. Gradually whisk in oil and season vinaigrette with salt and pepper.

jalapeno lime vinaigrette

Makes 1 cup
per tablespoon
Calories: 45
Protein: 0 g
Carbs: <1 g
Fat: 4 g
Sat: <1 g

1 2-inch fresh jalapeno chili
2/3 cup fresh lime juice
1 tablespoon rice wine vinegar
1/3 cup canola oil

In a blender combine the first three ingredients. With the motor running, add oil in a stream and blend 30 seconds or until emulsified.

raspberry vinaigrette

Serves 6
per portion
Calories: 50
Protein: <1 g
Carbs: 3 g
Fat: 5 g
Sat: 1 g

3/4 cup raspberry vinegar
1/3 cup chopped shallots
2 tablespoons extra-virgin olive oil
sea salt, white pepper

Blend vinegar and shallots in a blender or food processor. With the machine running, gradually add the oil and season with salt and pepper.

roasted pumpkin seed oil vinaigrette

I fell in love with this oil just for its radiant orange color,
then discovered the wonderful flavor it imparts to greens.
This type of oil tends to become bitter if heated, so it's best
not to use it for cooking.

1/4 cup fresh orange juice
2 tablespoons soy sauce
1 tablespoon plus 1 teaspoon roasted
    pumpkin seed oil
2 teaspoons white wine vinegar
1 teaspoon minced jalapeno chili
1 garlic clove, minced
1/2 teaspoon fresh, minced ginger
sea salt, pepper

Combine all the ingredients in a bowl and
refrigerate overnight. Serve at room temperature on
grilled shrimp or an avocado-tomato salad.

Serves 4
per portion
Calories: 54
Protein: 1 g
Carbs: 3 g
Fat: 5 g
Sat: <1 g

shallot vinaigrette

4 tablespoons extra-virgin olive oil
1/4 cup plus 2 tablespoons cider vinegar
2 shallots, minced
sea salt, pepper

In a small bowl, combine all the oil, vinegar and
shallots and season with taste with salt and pepper.
Bring to a boil on the stove and pour over greens,
such as baby spinach leaves.

Serves 8
per portion
Calories: 63
Protein: <1 g
Carbs: 1 g
Fat: 7 g
Sat: 1 g

I never drink—wine.
~Count Dracula~

sherry-mustard dressing

Serves 6
per portion
Calories: 65
Protein: <1 g
Carbs: 1 g
Fat: 7 g
Sat: 1 g

3 tablespoons chopped shallots
2 tablespoons sherry wine vinegar
1 teaspoon Dijon mustard
3 tablespoons extra-virgin olive oil

Whisk first three ingredients together in a medium bowl to blend. Gradually whisk in oil and season with sea salt and pepper to taste.

chipotle dressing

Serves 6
per portion
Calories: 67
Protein: <1 g
Carbs: 1 g
Fat: 7 g
Sat: 1 g

1/4 cup fresh orange juice
1 tablespoon finely chopped canned chipotle chilis
1/4 teaspoon ground cinnamon, preferably Mexican
1 teaspoon ground cumin
3 tablespoons extra-virgin olive oil

Whisk the first four ingredients together in a small bowl. Add the oil and whisk until blended.

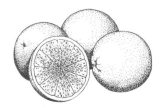

menomaise

My daughter jokingly referred to my creation as menomaise when she found it in the fridge. Real mayonnaise is made with soy oil but this version works nicely as a salad dressing, dip or sauce.

1/4 cup lemon juice
1/4 cup canola oil
4 teaspoons soy sauce
1/2 teaspoon sea salt
1/4 cup yellow onions, chopped
4 green onions, finely chopped
2 cloves garlic
1/3 cup chopped parsley
1/2 teaspoon curry powder
14 ounces tofu, drained and dried

per tablespoon
Calories: 38
Protein: 2 g
Carbs: 1 g
Fat: 3 g
Sat: 0 g

Place all the ingredients in a blender except the tofu and process.
Add the tofu and blend until smooth. Refrigerate overnight.
Makes 2 1/2 cups or 32 tablespoons.

menomaise for vegetables

1/4 cup lemon juice
1/4 cup canola oil
1 tablespoon dijon mustard
1 sprig fresh dill
1/2 teaspoon sea salt
14 ounces tofu, drained and dried

per tablespoon
Calories: 36
Protein: 2 g
Carbs: 1 g
Fat: 3 g
Sat: 0 g

Place all the ingredients in a blender except the tofu and process.
Add the tofu and blend until smooth. Refrigerate overnight.

chapter fourteen
dips, drinks and dairy

tuna dip

This is an updated version of an old recipe from Carlos N'
Charlie's, a celebrity hangout on the Sunset Strip in
Hollywood. Serve with fresh vegetables or scoop it into
romaine lettuce leaves.

Serves 10
per portion
(3 tablespoons)
Calories: 69
Protein: 10 g
Carbs: 0 g
Fat: 3 g
Sat: 1 g

1 12 1/2 ounce can tuna, drained
2 jalapeno chilis, seeded and stemmed
1 (1 inch) piece green onion (green part only)
1 (1 inch) piece celery
1/4 cup light mayonnaise
sea salt, pepper
4 leaves cilantro, chopped

Blend tuna, jalapenos, green onion and celery in
a food processor or blender (do not puree). Blend in
mayonnaise and seasoning. Blend to desired
consistency and sprinkle with cilantro.

It's all right to drink like a fish—
if you drink what a fish drinks.
~Mary Pettibone Poole~

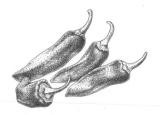

les tuillieres goat cheese and herb dip

Makes 1 1/2 cups
per tablespoon
Calories: 23
Protein: 1 g
Carbs: <1 g
Fat: 2 g
Sat: 1 g

In the town of Pont de Barret, near Nyons, France, I was served this delicious dip at Les Tuillieres, a lovely bed-and-breakfast. Add edible flowers for a special look.

6 ounces soft goat cheese
2 teaspoons extra-virgin olive oil
3 tablespoons yogurt, low fat
2 tablespoons chopped fresh chives
2 tablespoons chopped fresh Italian parsley
1 tablespoon chopped fresh cilantro
1 teaspoon chopped fresh mint
1 teaspoon chopped fresh thyme
1/2 teaspoon chopped fresh rosemary
1 tablespoon chopped assorted edible flowers

Blend goat cheese, oil and yogurt in the processor until smooth. Transfer to a small bowl and mix in all the herbs and flowers. Season dip to taste with salt and pepper. Cover and refrigerate until cold and flavors blend, about 3 hours.

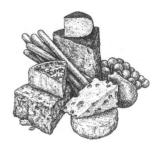

grilled zucchini and yogurt dip

2 medium zucchini (about 3/4 pound)
1 small garlic clove
1/2 teaspoon salt
1/4 cup plain, low-fat yogurt
2 teaspoons mayonnaise
1 tablespoon minced fresh spearmint leaves
1 teaspoon lemon juice

Serves 2
per 1/4 cup
Calories: 73
Protein: 3 g
Carbs: 6 g
Fat: 4 g
Sat: <1 g

Prepare grill.

Cut zucchini lengthwise into 1/4-inch thick slices and grill on an oiled rack set 5 to 6 inches over glowing coals until very tender, about 5 minutes on each side.

Mince garlic with salt and mash to a paste. Finely chop zucchini and stir into garlic paste with remaining ingredients.

Life is too short
to stuff a mushroom.
~Shirley Conrad~

grilled eggplant dip

Makes 3 cups
per 1/4 cup
Calories: 62
Protein: 1 g
Carbs: 6 g
Fat: 4 g
Sat: <1 g

This recipe needs to be prepared a day ahead of time, so I often make it for weekend get-togethers with my friends. Serve it in a hollowed-out eggplant for a special effect.

4 pounds medium eggplants
1 small red onion
2 large garlic cloves
2/3 cup packed fresh flat-leafed parsley leaves
2-2/3 tablespoons extra-virgin olive oil
3 tablespoons white-wine vinegar
2 tablespoons reduced-fat mayonnaise

Prepare grill.

Pierce eggplants in several places with a fork and grill on a rack set 5 to 6 inches over glowing coals, turning them occasionally, until very soft, 30 to 40 minutes. (If you don't want to prepare a grill, broil them about 6 inches from a preheated broiler for 30 to 40 minutes. The smoky flavor will be missing.)

Transfer eggplants to a colander and when cool enough to handle, quarter lengthwise. Remove as many seeds as possible. Scrape the flesh into a large sieve set over a bowl, discarding the skin. Drain eggplant, covered and chilled, 1 day. Discard any juices from the eggplant.

Mince onion and garlic and finely chop parsley. In a food processor pulse eggplant with onion, garlic, parsley and remaining ingredients until coarsely pureed. Transfer spread to a bowl and season with salt and pepper. Chill dip, covered at least 3 hours.

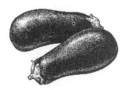

pinto bean and sun-dried tomato dip

1/2 cup boiling water
6 sun-dried tomato halves
　　(not packed in oil, about 1 ounce)
1 15-ounce can pinto beans, rinsed and drained
2 teaspoons extra-virgin olive oil
1 tablespoon red wine vinegar
1 teaspoon minced garlic
sea salt, pepper

Serves 6
per portion
Calories: 81
Protein: 4 g
Carbs: 13 g
Fat: 2 g
Sat: <1 g

　　Mix 1/2 cup boiling water and sun-dried tomatoes in a small bowl. Let stand until tomatoes soften, about 30 minutes. Drain; reserving soaking liquid. Chop tomatoes.
　　Finely chop tomaotes and beans in a processor. Blend in oil, vinegar and garlic. With machine running, gradually add 1/2 cup soaking liquid; puree. Season with sea salt and pepper.

tofu and veggies snack

2 ounces firm tofu
1/3 teaspoon olive oil
1/2 package dry onion soup mix

Serves 1
per portion
Calories: 113
Protein: 10 g
Carbs: 4 g
Fat: 7 g
Sat: 0 g

　　Place in blender until smooth. Refrigerate. Use with crisp vegetables for dipping.

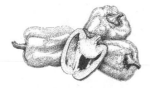

white bean hummus

Makes 3 cups
per tablespoon
Calories: 25
Protein: 1 g
Carbs: 4 g
Fat: 1 g
Sat: <1 g

This is a very low calorie version of a hummus without the tahini. Serve it sprinkled with Aleppo pepper for color and a unique, smoky flavor.

2 15-ounce cans navy beans
6 garlic cloves
2 tablespoons extra-virgin olive oil
1 teaspoon ground cumin
1/2 teaspoon ground coriander seeds
1/4 teaspoon salt
Pinch of cayenne

Rinse and drain beans. To a food processor with the motor running, drop garlic through the tube and blend until minced. Add beans and remaining ingredients and blend until smooth. Transfer to a serving bowl and chill, covered for 1 day. Just before serving sprinkle Aleppo pepper on top.

white bean dip with garlic, lemon and basil

Serves 4
per portion
(1/3 cup)
Calories: 52
Protein: 3 g
Carbs: 8 g
Fat: 1 g
Sat: 0 g

This is a great dip to keep on hand for snacks. It seems I never make enough.

4 cups white beans, soaked and cooked if dried,
    or straight from can (reserve any liquid)
1/3 cup coarsely chopped fresh basil or parsley leaves
1/4 cup lemon juice
1 tablespoon extra-virgin olive oil
2 large garlic cloves, crushed

Drain beans. Combine beans, basil, lemon juice, oil, and garlic in the bowl of a food processor. Process until smooth, adding reserved liquid tablespoon by tablespoon, as necessary. Add salt and pepper to taste. Refrigerate at least 1 hour.

Serve with crisp vegetables like peppers, celery, broccoli, daikon.

fourth of july cottage cheese

There is nothing faster than cottage cheese and fruit when you need to get out the door in a hurry. Berries lend a festive reminder of this holiday celebration, but don't substitute nonfat cottage cheese, as the fructose in the fruit will act like 3 tablespoons of corn syrup in your body.

1 cup 2% cottage cheese
1/4 cup blueberries
1/4 cup raspberries
1/4 cup strawberries

Serves 1
per portion
Calories: 227
Protein: 32 g
Carbs: 20 g
Fat: 5 g
Sat: 3 g

yogurt and nuts

This is another quick, easy snack to use.

1 cup low-fat yogurt
1 teaspoon slivered almonds

Serves 1
per portion
Calories: 161
Protein: 13 g
Carbs: 17 g
Fat: 5 g
Sat: 2 g

*Nobody can be insulted by
raspberries and cream.
~Barbara Kafka~*

black currant iced tea with cinnamon and ginger

Serves 8
per portion
Calories: 0
Protein: 0 g
Carbs: 0 g
Fat: 0 g
Sat: 0 g

I love iced teas and this one is especially pretty when served in a frosted glass with a little cinnamon stick.

6 cups water
12 wild black currant herbal tea bags
2 3-inch long cinnamon sticks, broken in half
1 tablespoon (packed) minced, peeled fresh ginger
Nutrasweet™

Bring 6 cups of water to boil in a large saucepan. Add tea bags, broken cinnamon sticks and fresh ginger. Remove from the heat; cover and steep 10 minutes. Chill until cold. Strain tea mixture into pitcher and sweeten with Nutrasweet™. Serve in frosted glasses with ice and garnish with cinnamon sticks.

Love and scandal
are the best sweeteners of tea.
~Henry Fielding~

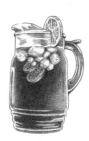

fruit toddy

This drink work equally well with raspberries, blackberries, boysenberries and blueberries. Be sure to get Ceylon cinnamon for a sweet taste, as other varieties will be too harsh and spoil the flavor.

Makes 1 cup
per cup
Calories: 20
Protein: <1 g
Carbs: 5 g
Fat: <1 g
Sat: 0 g

4 cups berries
3 cups bottled water
4 whole cloves
3 black peppercorns
3 cardamom pods, lightly crushed
2 Ceylon cinnamon sticks, broken into small pieces
1 bay leaf
Nutrasweet™

In a medium non-reactive saucepan, combine all the ingredients and bring to a boil. Cook over low heat for 30 minutes, gently crushing the berries against the side of the pan. Strain the berries through a fine sieve into a heat-proof bowl without pressing on the berries. Let cool. Stir in Nutrasweet™ before serving.

grapefruit coolers

Be sure and use the ruby grapefruit variety, which is packed with nutrients, in this refreshing drink.

Serves 12
per portion
Calories: 38
Protein: 1 g
Carbs: 10 g
Fat: 0 g
Sat: 0 g

9 cups fresh squeezed ruby grapefruit juice
(about 6 large grapefruits)
3 cups seltzer or club soda

In a pitcher half-filled with ice cubes stir together juice and seltzer or soda and garnish with mint.

herbed tomato juice

Serves 10
per portion
Calories: 37
Protein: 1 g
Carbs: 6 g
Fat: 1 g
Sat: <1 g

When tomatoes are in season, I love to make this liquified version of gazpacho and serve it in individual small, iced glass candle holders.

1 1/2 pounds ripe tomatoes, quartered
1 tablespoon extra-virgin olive oil
1 tablespoon plus 1 teaspoon red wine vinegar
2 teaspoons thyme leaves
2 teaspoons coarsely chopped tarragon
1 small garlic clove, minced
1 1/2 teaspoons sherry vinegar
Pinch of cayenne pepper
sea salt, white pepper

In a food processor combine the tomatoes, olive oil, red wine vinegar, thyme tarragon, garlic, sherry vinegar and cayenne and process until smooth. Season lightly with salt and black pepper. Transfer the puree to a bowl and refrigerate for at least 1 hour and up to 1 day.

Just before serving, strain the tomato juice through a fine sieve, pressing on the tomatoes. Season again with salt and pepper. Whisk until frothy, then pour into small cups and serve.

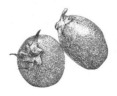

orangeade

6 cups fresh orange juice
4 1/2 cups chilled seltzer or club soda

    In a large pitcher stir together juice and seltzer or club soda and garnish with orange slices. Serve in tall glasses half-filled with ice.

Makes 10 cups
per cup
Calories: 67
Protein: 1 g
Carbs: 16 g
Fat: <1 g
Sat: 0 g

*All I ask of food is
that it doesn't harm me.
~ Michael Palin ~*

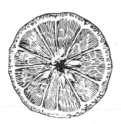

sassy rhubarb mint coolers

Serves 5
per portion
Calories: 19
Protein: 1 g
Carbs: 4 g
Fat: 0 g
Sat: 0 g

From April to June, the sassy stalks of rhubarb wave at me from the produce section, inviting me to drink in their luscious color. Long considered a spring tonic for its medicinal properties, rhubarb is really a vegetable that is painfully tart. Try this cooler topped with a jaunty hat of mint for a real change!

1 pound trimmed rhubarb
1 teaspoon anise seeds
5 cups water
1/4 cup packed fresh mint leaves
Nutrasweet™

Cut rhubarb into 1/2-inch pieces and in a saucepan bring to a boil with water, anise and mint leaves. Simmer mixture, stirring occasionally, 15 minutes (rhubarb will disintegrate) and cool 15 minutes. Pour mixture through a fine sieve into a pitcher, pressing hard on solids. Chill mixture, covered, until cold, about 3 hours. Add Nutrasweet™ to taste only when thoroughly chilled.

Serve coolers over ice in glasses garnished with mint sprigs.

You have to eat normal
or you'll dry up.
Anybody knows that.
~Kay Thompson~

smoky "virgin" mary

Be sure and use a vegetable or tomato juice that doesn't have any added corn syrup.

3 cups vegetable juice
2 tablespoons fresh lemon juice
1 tablespoon minced fresh cilantro
1 tablespoon Worcestershire sauce
1 teaspoon finely minced, seeded, canned chipotle chilies
1 teaspoon ground cumin
6 stalks celery with leafy tops for garnish

Mix everything but the celery in a pitcher and chill until cold, at least 2 hours or overnight.
Fill 6 tall glasses with ice and pour mixture over it. Garnish with the celery stalks.

Serves 6
per portion
Calories: 26
Protein: 1 g
Carbs: 6 g
Fat: 0 g
Sat: 0 g

sparkling berry lemonade

Use whatever berries are in season for this delicious, cooling drink.

3 cups quartered fresh berries (strawberries,
    blueberries, blackberries, raspberries)
12 ounces fresh squeezed lemon juice
3 cups sparkling water, chilled
6 packets Nutrasweet™

Combine strawberries and lemon juice in a blender and process until smooth.
Add sparkling water and Nutrasweet; pour over ice.

Serves 6
1 cup serving
Calories: 35
Protein: 1 g
Carbs: 9 g
Fat: <1 g
Sat: 0 g

appendix a
resources for
healthy living

the menopause diet website

If you are interested in learning more about the impact of diet on menopause, visit my website at

www.menopausediet.com

where you will find up to date news articles, discussions about the latest scientific research, a newsletter just for menopausal women and products of interest to us. You can order personally autographed copies online of "The Menopause Diet," "The Menopause Diet Mini Meal Cookbook," "The Menopause Diet Daily Journal," motivational audio tapes along with my nutritional supplements "Female Formula Stress Tabs" and "Pyridoxal-5 Phosphate" or by calling

1-800-554-3335 in the United States
or
310 471-2375
if you do not have access to the Internet.

Share your personal experience with The Menopause Diet Plan on my message board and swap recipes and support with each other. It can be just the helping hand you need!

female formula stress tabs
60 tablets

Two tablets contain:

Beta Carotene	5000 i.u.
D-alpha Tocopherol Acetate	200 i.u.
Sodium Selenite	83 mcg
Zinc Gluconate	35 mg
Vit. C (from ascorbyl palmitate and ascorbic acid)	350 mg
Calcium Carbonate	750 mg
Magnesium Hydroxide	360 mg
Vit. D3 (cholecalciferol)	33 i.u.
Biotin	33 mcg
D-Calcium Pantothenate	166 mg
Riboflavin	66 mg
Potassium Chloride	50 mg
Chromium (amino acid chelate)	83 mcg
Manganese Gluconate	41 mg

pyridoxal-5-phosphate
30 tablets

One tablet contains:

Pyridoxal-5-Phosphate (enteric coated)	20mg

All supplements are 100% natural and free of yeast, corn, sugar, starch, soy, flavors, colors, preservatives, wheat or milk derivatives. All orders are shipped Priority Mail.

nutridata software

The nutritional analysis of the recipes in this cookbook was performed using Nutridata Software's Cooking Companion and Diet Balancer programs. Rated the best by SHAPE magazine, these programs share information, putting complete nutrient data at your fingertips while easily adjusting for special diets like The Menopause Diet. The Cooking Companion prints out a shopping list and The Diet Balancer even includes exercise calories in calculating your nutritional requirements. Both programs are available for $39 each at major retail stores. A computer version of "The Menopause Diet Mini Meal Cookbook" that works with your Nutridata Software, is available. You can obtain both programs and the cookbook disc by calling

1-800-554-3335
or by contacting my website
http://www.menopausediet.com

spices

Purchasing new, exotic spices can lend a real zip to foods while keeping the fat low. One of the best sources is Penzeys Spice catalog. You can order their catalog online at:
• Penzeys Spices
www.penzeys.com
414 679-7207.

For Aleppo, pasilla and ancho chili powder, Dean and Deluca is an excellent resource. You can order online at:
• Dean and Deluca
www.dean-deluca-napavalley.com
707 967-9880.

Other sources for exotic spices are:
- Kalustyan
123 Lexington Ave
New York, NY 10016
212 685-3451

This mail order store has the most unusual ingredients for making traditional Indian dishes. They are a good source for curry leaves, fenugreek seeds, black or brown mustard seeds and tamarind concentrate.
- Sultan's Delight
P.O. Box 090302
Brooklyn, NY 11209
800 852-6844
718 745-6844
Fax 718 745-2563

- The Spice House
1031 N. Old World Third St
Milwaukee, WI 53203
414 272-0977

An excellent source for asian spices, such as chinese brown bean paste, star anise, fish sauce, chile paste.
- Uwajimaya
800 889-1928

Sadaf brand pomegranate paste for Middle Eastern dishes.
- Foods of India
212 683-4419

Dried New Mexican red chilies
- Chile Today-Hot Tamale
800 468-7377

A great source for banana leaves and dried ancho chilies if you don't have a Latino shop nearby.
- Kitchen Market
212 243-4433

This store will ship fresh curry leaves, tamarind concentrate, dried pomegrante seeds and brown mustard seeds.
- Adriana's Caravan
409 Vanderbilt St
Brooklyn, NY 11218
718 436-8565

Kaboucha squash, chilies and wax peppers can be found at this unique supplier.
- Frieda's
P.O. Box 58488
Los Angeles, CA 90058
800 241-1771
http://www.friedas.com

Sweet Spanish smoked paprika.
- La Tienda
http://www.tienda.com

- The Spanish Table
206 682-2827

teas

One of my favorite teas is made by Bernardaud's of France. It's a caramel tea and is rich in flavor, even when laced with a little milk You can order it from:
- La Cucina Rustica
cyberbaskets.com/cbdocs/items/be9003c.htm
9950 West Lawrence Avenue, Suite 202
Schiller Park, IL 60176 USA
800 796-0116 – Customer Service Department

Stash makes a Mango Passion Fruit tea available in

grocery stores and Ceylon Passion has a delightful
Passion Fruit Papaya tea combination. A mixture of
black teas with fruit extract, they make delightful iced
teas. All are caffeine free and available in your grocery
store.

Tejava is a delicious micro brewed tea made
entirely from the top two leaves of each branch
picked only from May through October. If you can't
find it in your grocery store, call 1-800-4-GEYSER.

tomatoes

There is nothing better than fresh tomatoes, but
the organic canned tomatoes seasoned with sea salt
by Muir Glen do well in a pinch. If you don't find
them in your grocery store, call or write
• Muir Glen
P.O. Box 1498
Sacramento, CA
707 778-7801
www.muirglen.com has a store locator on the site.

sea salt

Searching for specialty sea salts has become a hobby
of mine and I will share with you my secret sources.

This company sells Maldon Crystal sea salt, Celtic
Grey and Fleur de sel de Guaerande, the most expensive
type of salt, harvested under special conditions.
• The Baker's Catalog
P.O. Box 876
Norwich, VT 05055-0876
800 827-6836

This is another source for Fleur de sel de
Guerande.
• Zingerman's
422 Detroit St.
Ann Arbor, MI 48104
888 636-8162

This company carries Sicilian sea salt and Japanese Oshima Island salt.
• Corti Brothers
5810 Folsom Blvd.
Sacramento, CA 95822
800 509-FOOD

the greatest grater

Microplane has found a new use for a woodworker's rasp—zesting citrus, cheese and chocolate. These blades come in fine or coarse ratings which can be simply changed out as needed. You can purchase them from Sur La Table or from Microplane for under $15.
• Microplane
Lee Valley Tools
800 871-8158

japanese mandolin

This nifty little device is like an apple corer only standing upright. It can make oodles of noodles out of any hard vegetable with just a turn of the handle. You can purchase one called a Saladacco from Sur La Table for $35.95.
• Sur La Table
800 243-0842

chocolate soap

I'm all in a lather over this find! Fleurs de Chocolat has bath products composed of cocoa extract, pear and orange essences that could send Casanova into a swoon. I adore their Chocolate soap.
• Fleurs de Chocolat
800 373-7420

But when you want a bite of the real thing, try:
• Scharffen Berger Chocolate
250 S. Maple Ave., Unit C
S. San Francisco, CA 94080
800 930-4528
http://www.scharffen-berger.com

The primary requisite for
writing well about food
is a good appetite.
~ A.J. Liebling ~

appendix b

references

1. US Department of Health and Human Services, P.H.S., Centers for Disease Control and Prevention, National Center for Health Statistics, *Death and death rates for the 10 leading causes of death in specified age groups, by race and sex: US 1996.* National Vital Statistics Report, 1998. **47**(9): p. 29, 32, 36, 64-65.

2. Gannon, M. and F. Nuttall, *Factors affecting interpretation of postprandial glucose and insulin areas.* Diabetes Care, 1987. **10**: p. 759-763.

3. Melanson, K., et al., *Blood glucose and hormonal response to small and large meals in healthy young and old women.* J Gerontol: Biol Sc, 1998. **53A**: p. 4.

4. Wolever, T.M., *The glycemic index.* World Rev Nutr Diet, 1990. **62**: p. 120-85.

5. Ludwig, D.S., et al., *High glycemic index foods, overeating, and obesity.* Pediatrics, 1999. **103**(3): p. E26.

6. Michnovicz, J., *Environmental modulation of oestrogen metabolism in humans.* Int Clin Nutr Rev, 1987. **7**: p. 169-173.

7. Bucala, R., et al., *Increased levels of 16 alpha-hydroxyestrone-modified proteins in pregnancy and in systemic lupus erythematosus.* J Clin Endocrinol Metab, 1985. **60**(5): p. 841-7.

8. Fishman, J., J. Schneider, and R.e.a. Hershcopf, *Increased estrogen 16alpha-hydroxylase activity in women with breast and endometrial cancer.* J Steroid Biochem, 1984. **20**: p. 1077-1081.

9. Anderson, K.E., et al., *The influence of dietary protein and carbohydrate on the principal oxidative biotransformations of estradiol in normal subjects.* J Clin Endocrinol Metab, 1984. **59**(1): p. 103-7.

10. Longcope, C., et al., *The effect of a low fat diet on estrogen metabolism.* J Clin Endocrinol Metab, 1987. **64**(6): p. 1246-50.

11. Pomerleau, J., et al., *Effect of protein intake on glycaemic control and renal function in type 2 (non-insulin-dependent) diabetes mellitus.* Diabetologia, 1993. **36**(9): p. 829-34.

12. Preuss, H.G., et al., *Effects of diets high in refined carbohydrates on renal ammonium excretion in rats.* Am J Physiol, 1986. **250**(2 Pt 1): p. E156-63.

13. Reyes, A.A. and S. Klahr, *Dietary supplementation of L-arginine ameliorates renal hypertrophy in rats fed a high-protein diet.* Proc Soc Exp Biol Med, 1994. **206**(2): p. 157-61.

14. Fields, C.E. and R.G. Makhoul, *Vasomotor tone and the role of nitric oxide.* Semin Vasc Surg, 1998. **11**(3): p. 181-92.

15. Barzel, U.S. and L.K. Massey, *Excess dietary protein can adversely affect bone.* J Nutr, 1998. **128**(6): p. 1051-3.

16. Sharma, R.D., T.C. Raghuram, and N.S. Rao, *Effect of fenugreek seeds on blood glucose and serum lipids in type I diabetes.* Eur J Clin Nutr, 1990. **44**(4): p. 301-6.

17. Khan, A., et al., *Insulin potentiating factor and*

chromium content of selected foods and spices. Biol Trace Elem Res, 1990. **24**(3): p. 183-8.

18. Wolever, T.M. and J.B. Miller, *Sugars and blood glucose control.* Am J Clin Nutr, 1995. **62**(1 Suppl): p. 212S-221S; discussion 221S-227S.

19. Gonzalez Vilchez, F., et al., *Cardiac manifestations of primary hypothyroidism. Determinant factors and treatment response.* Rev Esp Cardiol, 1998. **51**(11): p. 893-900.

20. Nunez, S. and J. Leclere, *Diagnosis of hypothyroidism in the adult.* Rev Prat, 1998. **48**(18): p. 1993-8.

21. Massoudi, M.S., et al., *Prevalence of thyroid antibodies among healthy middle-aged women.* Findings from the thyroid study in healthy women. Ann Epidemiol, 1995. **5**(3): p. 229-33.

22. Reinhardt, W., et al., *Effect of small doses of iodine on thyroid function in patients with Hashimoto's thyroiditis residing in an area of mild iodine deficiency [see comments].* Eur J Endocrinol, 1998. **139**(1): p. 23-8.

23. Konno, N., et al., *Association between dietary iodine intake and prevalence of subclinical hypothyroidism in the coastal regions of Japan.* J Clin Endocrinol Metab, 1994. **78**(2): p. 393-7.

24. Chen, Y.D., et al., *Why do low-fat high-carbohydrate diets accentuate postprandial lipemia in patients with NIDDM?* Diabetes Care, 1995. **18**(1): p. 10-6.

25. Ginsberg, H.N., et al., *Increases in dietary cholesterol are associated with modest increases in both LDL and HDL cholesterol in healthy young women.* Arterioscler Thromb Vasc Biol, 1995. **15**(2): p. 169-78.

26. Jiang, Y.H., R.B. McGeachin, and C.A. Bailey,

alpha-tocopherol, beta-carotene, and retinol enrichment of chicken eggs. Poult Sci, 1994. **73**(7): p. 1137-43.

27. Kris-Etherton, P.M., et al., *The role of fatty acid saturation on plasma lipids, lipoproteins, and apolipoproteins: I. Effects of whole food diets high in cocoa butter, olive oil, soybean oil, dairy butter, and milk chocolate on the plasma lipids of young men [see comments].* Metabolism, 1993. **42**(1): p. 121-9.

28. Miller, J. and T. Leeds, *The G.I. Factor: The Glycaemic Index Solution.* 1996: Hodder Healine Asutralia Pty. Ltd.

29. Lewis, S.J., et al., *Lower serum oestrogen concentrations associated with faster intestinal transit.* Br J Cancer, 1997. **76**(3): p. 395-400.

30. Melanson, K.J., et al., *The effects of age on postprandial thermogenesis at four graded energetic challenges: findings in young and older women.* J Gerontol A Biol Sci Med Sci, 1998. **53**(6): p. B409-14.

index

order form

Give the gift of great health to your loved ones, friends and colleagues
Check your leading bookstore or order here

fax orders:	**telephone orders:**	**e-mail orders:**	**postal orders:**
(310) 471-9041.	Call	orders@	Healthy Life
(please send a	1-(800) 554-3335	menopausediet.	Publications,
copy of this form)	toll free or	com	264 South
	(310) 471-2375 if		La Cienega Blvd.,
	outside the United		PMB #1233,
	States and Canada.		Beverly Hills,
	Have your		California 90211
	credit card ready.		USA

Please send _____ copies of *The Menopause Diet* at $17.95 plus $4 shipping per book in the United States (California residents please add $1.48 sales tax per book). Canadian orders must be accompanied by a postal order in U.S. funds. International orders add $9 for shipping.

Please send me information on your other products _____

If you would like to order Female Formula Stress Tabs, Pyridoxal-5-Phosphate or the *Menopause Diet Daily Journal*, call 1-800-554-3335 24 hours a day. Operators are waiting for your call.

My check or money order for $_____ is enclosed.
United States $21.95 (outside of California)
                  $23.43 (within California)
Canada $25.00 (US funds)
International $27.00 (US funds)

Please charge my   VISA   MC

Name: _____

Address: _____

City: _____ State: _____ Zip: _____

Phone: _____ E-mail: _____

Card #: _____ Exp date: _____

Signature: _____

Please make your check payable and return to:
Healthy Life Publications
264 S. La Cienega Blvd., PMB #1233, Beverly Hills, California 90211
CALL YOUR CREDIT CARD ORDER TO: 800-554-3335
Fax: 310-471-9041 e-mail: orders@menopausediet.com

order form

Give the gift of great health to your loved ones, friends and colleagues
Check your leading bookstore or order here

fax orders:	telephone orders:	e-mail orders:	postal orders:
(310) 471-9041.	Call	orders@	Healthy Life
(please send a	1-(800) 554-3335	menopausediet.	Publications,
copy of this form)	toll free or	com	264 South
	(310) 471-2375 if		La Cienega Blvd.,
	outside the United		PMB #1233,
	States and Canada.		Beverly Hills,
	Have your		California 90211
	credit card ready.		USA

Please send _____ copies of *The Menopause Diet* at $17.95 plus $4 shipping per book in the United States (California residents please add $1.48 sales tax per book). Canadian orders must be accompanied by a postal order in U.S. funds. International orders add $9 for shipping.

Please send me information on your other products _____

If you would like to order Female Formula Stress Tabs, Pyridoxal-5-Phosphate or the *Menopause Diet Daily Journal*, call 1-800-554-3335 24 hours a day. Operators are waiting for your call.

My check or money order for $_____ is enclosed.
United States $21.95 (outside of California)
                   $23.43 (within California)
Canada $25.00 (US funds)
International $27.00 (US funds)

Please charge my   VISA   MC

Name: _____

Address: _____

City: _____ State: _____ Zip: _____

Phone: _____ E-mail: _____

Card #: _____ Exp date: _____

Signature: _____

Please make your check payable and return to:
Healthy Life Publications
264 S. La Cienega Blvd., PMB #1233, Beverly Hills, California 90211
CALL YOUR CREDIT CARD ORDER TO: 800-554-3335
Fax: 310-471-9041 e-mail: orders@menopausediet.com

order form

Give the gift of great health to your loved ones, friends and colleagues
Check your leading bookstore or order here

fax orders:	**telephone orders:**	**e-mail orders:**	**postal orders:**
(310) 471-9041.	Call	orders@	Healthy Life
(please send a	1-(800) 554-3335	menopausediet.	Publications,
copy of this form)	toll free or	com	264 South
	(310) 471-2375 if		La Cienega Blvd.,
	outside the United		PMB #1233,
	States and Canada.		Beverly Hills,
	Have your		California 90211
	credit card ready.		USA

Please send _____ copies of *The Menopause Diet* at $17.95 plus $4 shipping per book in the United States (California residents please add $1.48 sales tax per book). Canadian orders must be accompanied by a postal order in U.S. funds. International orders add $9 for shipping.

Please send me information on your other products _____

If you would like to order Female Formula Stress Tabs, Pyridoxal-5-Phosphate or the *Menopause Diet Daily Journal*, call 1-800-554-3335 24 hours a day. Operators are waiting for your call.

My check or money order for $_____ is enclosed.
United States $21.95 (outside of California)
                 $23.43 (within California)
Canada $25.00 (US funds)
International $27.00 (US funds)

Please charge my   VISA   MC

Name: _____

Address: _____

City: _____ State: _____ Zip: _____

Phone: _____ E-mail: _____

Card #: _____ Exp date: _____

Signature: _____

Please make your check payable and return to:
Healthy Life Publications
264 S. La Cienega Blvd., PMB #1233, Beverly Hills, California 90211
CALL YOUR CREDIT CARD ORDER TO: 800-554-3335
Fax: 310-471-9041 e-mail: orders@menopausediet.com